I0082620

To 'Air' is Human

Everything You Ever Wanted to Know About Intestinal Gas

Volume Two

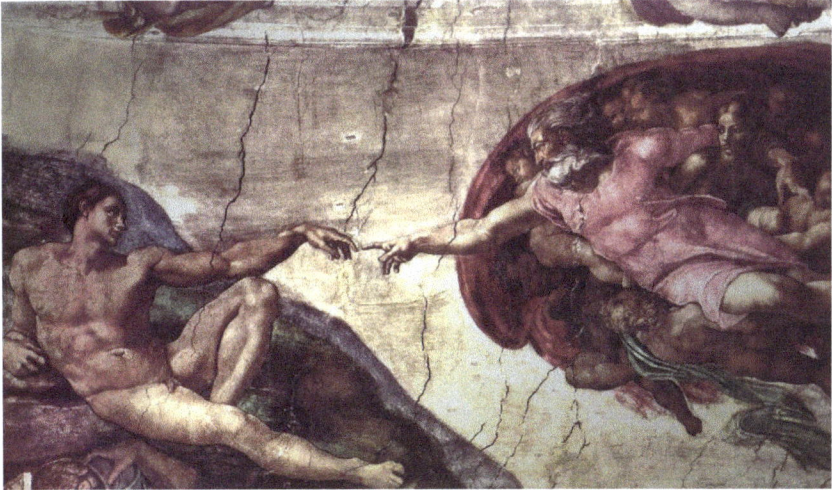

Joseph B. Weiss, MD, FACP, FACG, AGAF
Clinical Professor of Medicine,
Gastroenterology
University of California, San Diego

© 2016 Joseph B. Weiss, M.D.
SmartAsk Books
Rancho Santa Fe, California, USA
www.smartaskbooks.com

All rights reserved. No part of the text of this book may be reproduced, reused, republished, or retransmitted in any form, or stored in a database or retrieval system, without written permission of the publisher.

ISBN-13: 978-1-943760-14-5 (Color - Volume One)
ISBN-13: 978-1-943760-15-2 (Color - Volume Two)
ISBN-13: 978-1-943760-02-2 (Color – Combined Volumes)

Last digit is the print number: 9 8 7 6 5 4 3

Dedication

This volume is dedicated to clearing the air of the misperception that intestinal gas is anything other than a normal physiologic process common to all humanity. Nature and natural processes should be universally accepted as one of the cherished principles of fundamental human rights.

I am indebted to my loved ones Nancy, Danielle, Jeremy, Courie, Lizzy, & Indy. They have offered their insights, suggestions, comments, and unwavering support throughout the long process of having this project finally come to pass. You will always be the mighty wind beneath my wings.

Table of Contents - Volume One

Introduction

Intestinal gas has been generated and released by every human who has ever lived Very few people understand the underlying physiology of its generation or the law of physics, which play an important part in our experience of this universal condition. **To 'Air' is Human, Everything You Ever Wanted to Know About Intest** **Gas** is an informative, entertaining, and understandable volume designed to enlighten the lay public with everything they may have ever wanted to know about intestinal gas, but were too embarrassed to ask. Because of its size, over ninety tho words, and more than three hundred pages with hundreds of images, the electroni is the best value as the expense of color printing is substantial. A more economical version with a non-color interior is available.

The word fart is the correct word to use in the English language, and indeed is one it's oldest words. The alternative terms used, such as flatus and flatulence are not original English words as they have been borrowed from the Latin. There is controversy as to the derivation of the word fart. It is thought to have Indo-Europe roots in the Germanic language word farzen. One thought is that it originated as an onomatopoeia, a word that phonetically imitates the sound of the event it describe Another thought is that it was related to the term for partridge, as the bird makes a similar sound when it is disturbed in its natural habitat and takes flight.

Farts are ubiquitous, all living creatures generate gas from cellular metabolism and respiration, and humans are no exception. The bacteria of your colonic flora, part c the microbiome of living organisms that lives on and within humans, generate gas which collect in the bowel. They are joined with the air swallowed throughout the day and night, particularly at meals.

Aerophagia is universal and we swallow on average three to five cubic centimeters (one teaspoonful) of air with every swallow. Additional gasses are produced durin; the enzymatic digestive processes as well as the neutralization of gastric hydrochloric acid by pancreatic and duodenal bicarbonate. The result is a significa: volume of gasses within and transiting the bowel.

Fortunately the vast majority of the gasses produced are absorbed by the gut, then into the bloodstream through diffusion and finally exhaled when they each th alveoli of the lungs. The component gasses have very different properties of diffusion through the bowel wall and into the bloodstream. Carbon dioxide readily diffuses and enters solution and is exhaled promptly. Although it is the largest volume of gas generated, and temporarily contributes to distension and postprand (after meal) discomfort, it is the easiest to eliminate from the bowel and is only a minor contributor to flatulence.

The volume of gasses in the gastrointestinal tract is dependent on the quantity and nature of foods ingested, the body's ability to produce enzymes for the various foo types, the microbiome and gut flora, and gastrointestinal transit time. The often quoted figure of twelve farts per day is a reasonable average number of farts passe but there is a very wide range of what is considered normal.

Continued from Volume One

Fart, Therapeutic Options

Many individuals have issues with unpleasant fecal odors, and unfortunately it is not as easily remedied as flushing or walking away. The fecal aroma generated by the gut microbiome that smells in defecated feces is the identical aroma that may be discharged with intestinal gas, fecal incontinence, fistula, ostomies, diarrhea, inflammatory bowel disease, after gastric bypass surgery, and a host of other conditions. The numbers of individuals affected is in the millions in the United States alone. Unfortunately, the majority of the general public remains uninformed and impose a social stigma on a medical condition over which they have limited or no control.

Fortunately there are a number of effective therapeutic options available, but too many sufferers are not aware of or have access to them. They range from external appliances and clothing, to external and internal deodorants and suppressants. Of course there are also tongue-in-cheek suggestions ,such as getting a dog to blame as the source of the fart odor. The Merck Manual a few years back suggested working on perfecting one's glare, just glare at someone else as if they were the source.

More direct references to farts has been employed in the advertising campaign of air-freshener company Poo-Pourri. Although the advertising campaign received a nomination as one of the worst ads by a national newspaper, it was a major hit on social media with over thirty million views. For a holiday themed advertisement Santa Claus is farting on the toilet while an attractive model sings a parody of a seasonal tune.

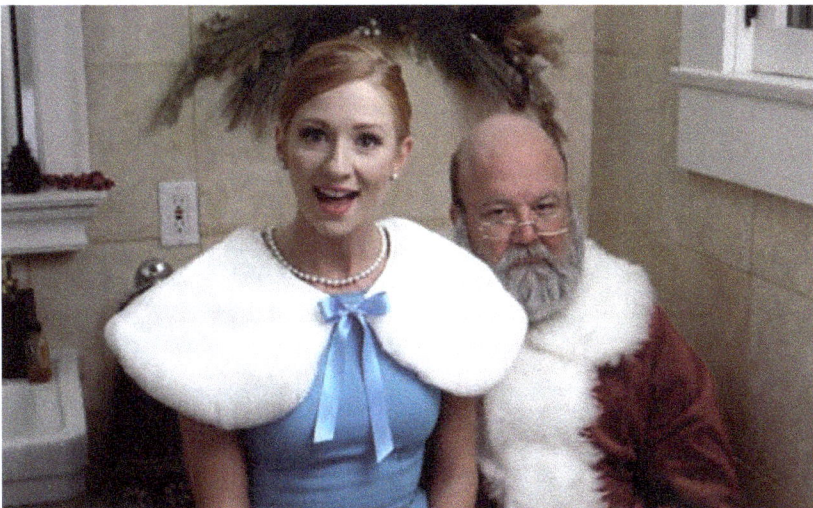

Poo-Pourri Advertising video www.ninjamarkweting.it

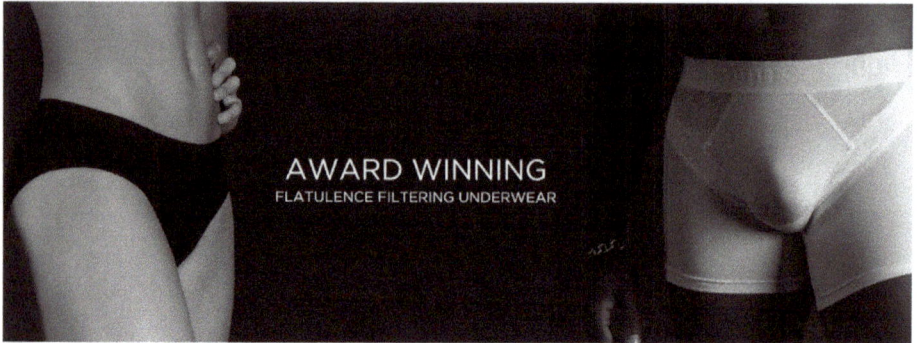

Shreddies advertising campaign for activated charcoal odor adsorbing underwear myshreddies.com

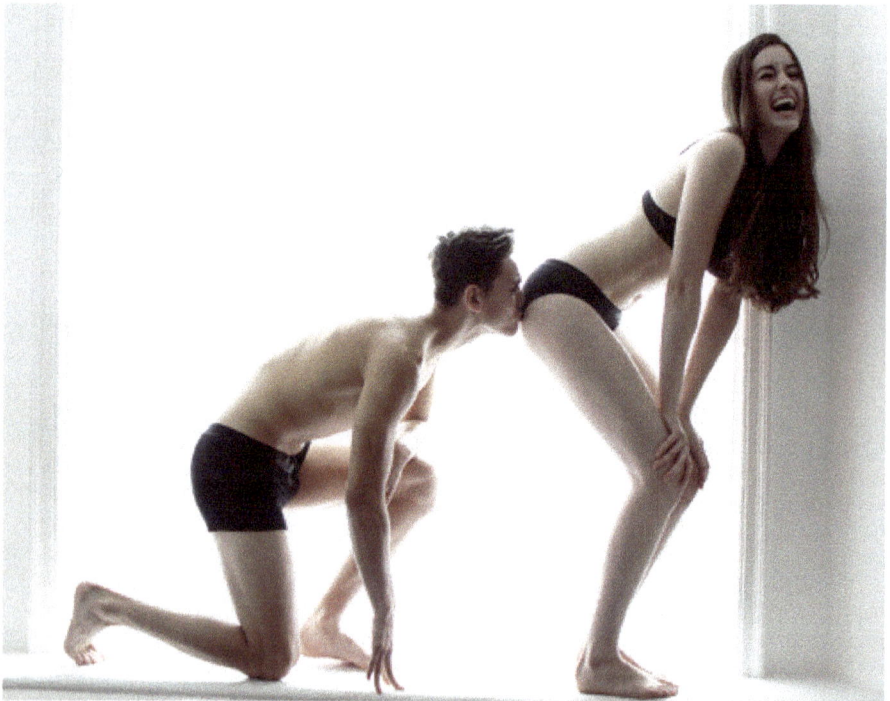

Shreddies advertising campaign for activated charcoal odor adsorbing underwear myshreddies.com

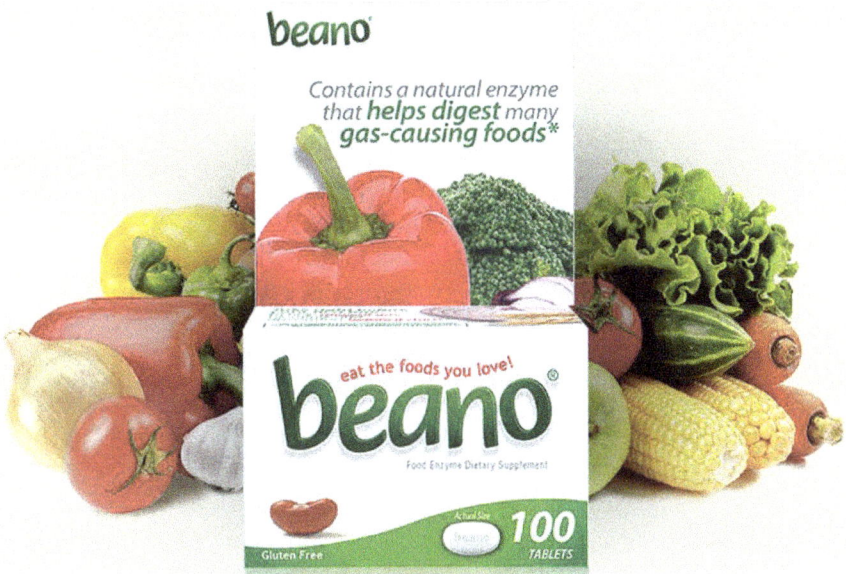

Beano was one of the first products to advertise a product designed to reduce intestinal gas. Its ad first appeared in Vegetarian Times

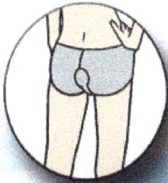
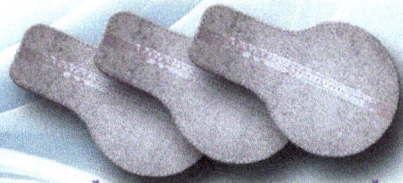
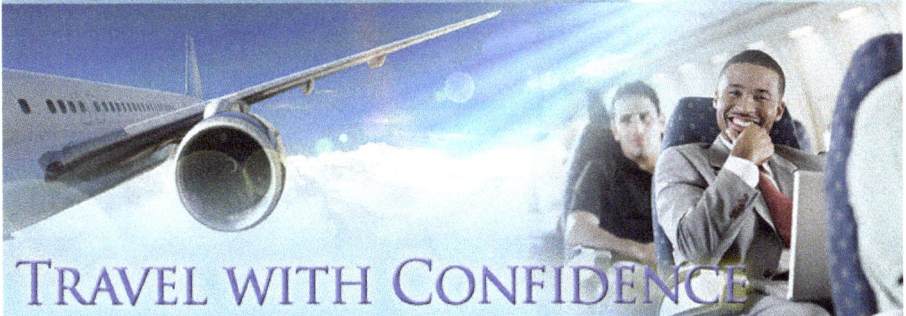

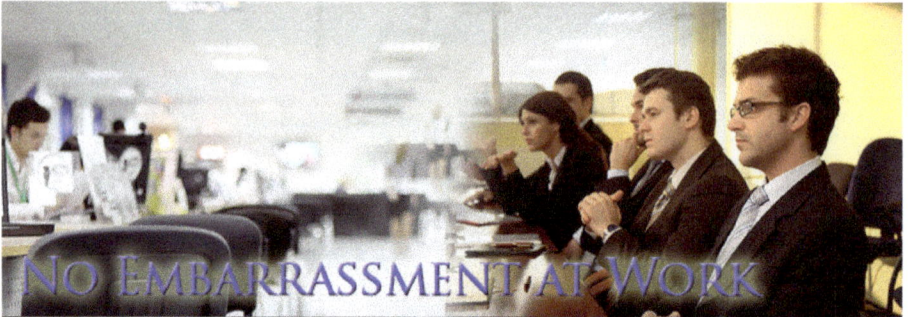

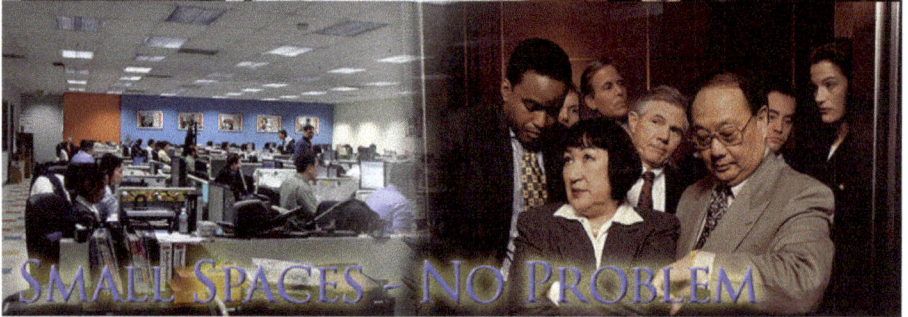

Flat-D advertises and markets a wide variety of activated charcoal products to adsorb the aroma of flatus and other body odors. www.flat-d.com

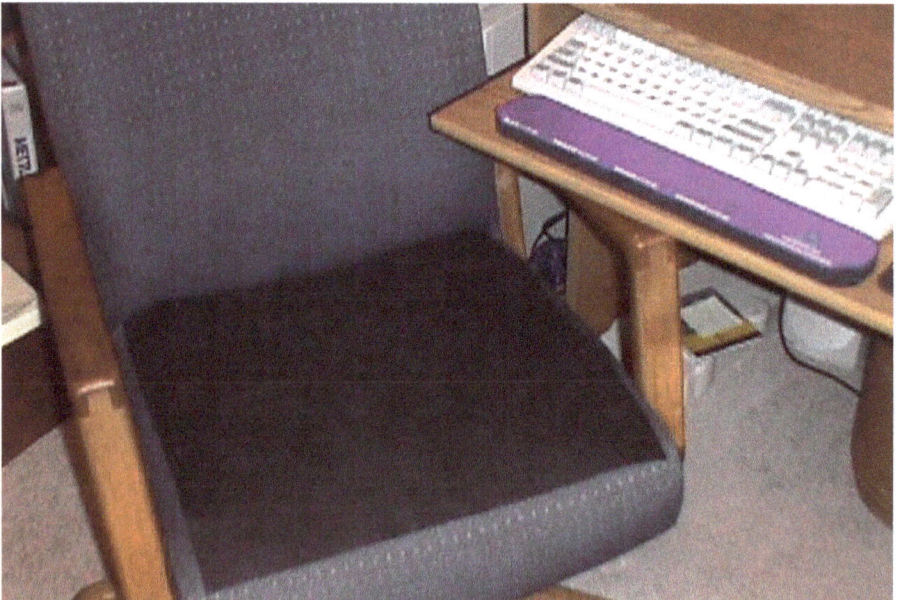

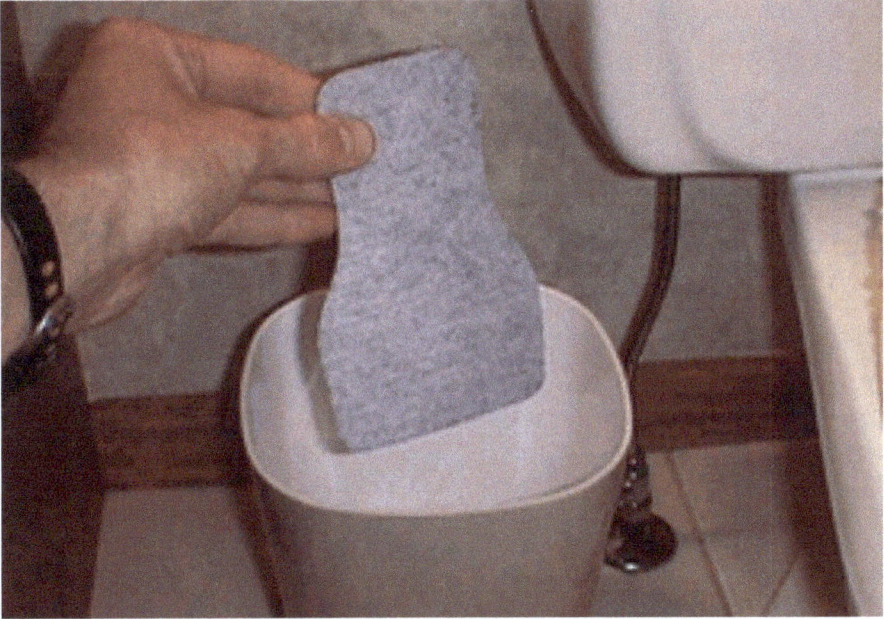

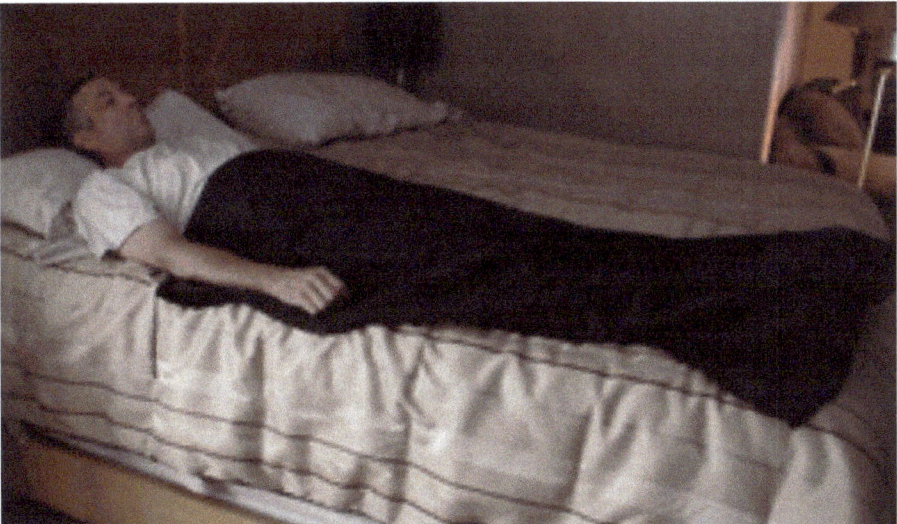

Flat-D advertises and markets a wide variety of activated charcoal products to adsorb the aroma of flatus and other body odors. Activated charcoal seat cushions, liners for underwear and clothing, and sleeping sack are amongst the numerous products they offer. www.flat-d.com

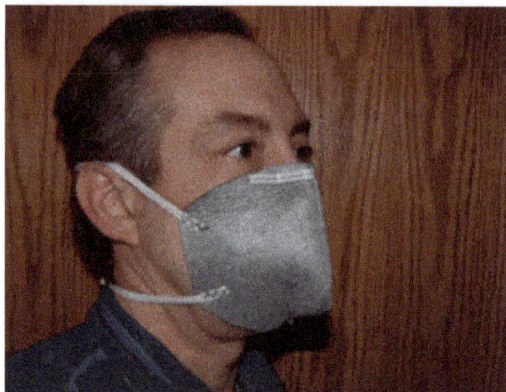

Flat-D offers another approach to protect the individual from offensive odors, by wearing an activated charcoal facemask covering the mouth and nose. www.flat-d.com

Surprisingly where it can provide relief and comfort to many sufferers, some media outlets refuse to place advertisements for products dealing with flatulence and ostomy odors. Deodorants, feminine hygiene douches, tampons, sanitary napkins for menstruation, diapers for adults with incontinence, erectile dysfunction prescriptions, etcetera have been seen by the public and the country still stands. Devrom, an effective internal deodorant that suppresses fecal odor was not allowed to place their advertisement in Reader's Digest or AARP (Association for the Advancement of Retired People) because it contained the word stool and smelt flatulence. Somehow the publications did not see the irony in that their policy did not pass the smell test.

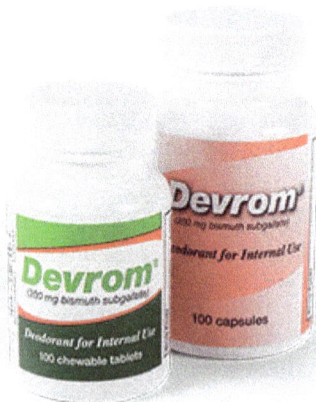

Devrom is an over the counter preparation of bismuth subgallate and has been marketed for over fifty years as an internal deodorant. Bismuth does have antibacterial properties it may change the microbiome by reducing the organisms that contribute to offensive flatulence. Another bismuth product that has been popular in the marketplace is Pepto-Bismol, which is a bismuth subsalicylate. Bismuth subsalicylate is related to aspirin (salicylic acid) and does not appear to provide as significant relief from the unpleasant odors as has been reported with Devrom.

To 'Air' is Human Volume Two

It has been particularly popular for individuals who have undergone gastric bypass surgery, inflammatory bowel disease, as well as those with ostomies, and others. With advances in surgery, and the ability to preserve sphincters or create artificial sphincters, ostomies are seen less frequently. This is where the intestinal discharge exits the body through an artificial opening, the ostomy, created at surgery. Because the bowel is diverted from the colon less moisture is absorbed and the feces may be semi-formed or liquid.

The more liquid form allows for the more rapid vaporization of volatile organic compounds and gasses that give rise to the feculent odor. In spite of being in otherwise excellent health, many individuals with these issues find themselves socially restricted in their activities because of concern about embarrassment or offending others. Safe and effective products are available, but many individuals are unaware and suffer unnecessarily because of the lack of information and understanding.

Bismuth is a chemical element, number eighty-three on the periodic table, which has long history of being used in preparations designed to treat gastrointestinal complaints. It is a heavy metal with a low level of toxicity. Its various compound have also been used historically to treat syphilis and the severe diarrhea from cholera. Bismuthinite is a mineral consisting of bismuth sulfide (Bi_2S_3) and is an important ore for bismuth.

The mechanism of action is unknown and may be related to its known antimicrobial activity, perhaps inhibiting the microbes that generate some of the more offensive gasses that are usually contain sulfur as well as aromatic and volatile organic compounds. Bismuth also reacts directly with sulfur generating bismuth sulfide, a dark black insoluble compound. This can cause darkening or blackening of the tongue if sulfur is found in high concentrations in the saliva. It will also cause blackening of the stool as it binds with the sulfur that would otherwise give rise to hydrogen sulfide and other offensive sulfur gasses. The dark black color of the stool may be mistaken for melena, a sign of internal bleeding that results from the digestive process on blood cells and hemoglobin. The black coloration is not a health concern and is temporary clearing with cessation of bismuth intake.

Activated carbon is used to treat oral poisonings by binding to and preventing the poison from being absorbed by the gastrointestinal tract. Charcoal biscuits were marketed in the early 19th century as an antidote to flatulence, and are still marketed today for diarrhea, indigestion, flatulence, and as a pet care product. Unfortunately orally ingested charcoal pills are not effective in appreciably reducing intestinal gas. This may be because the adsorptive capacity of the activated charcoal is fully utilized before it finally gets to the colon where its gas adsorbing properties are needed. Fortunately, bismuth products do provide a significant advantage by binding to the sulfur compounds and eliminating them without producing offensive gas.

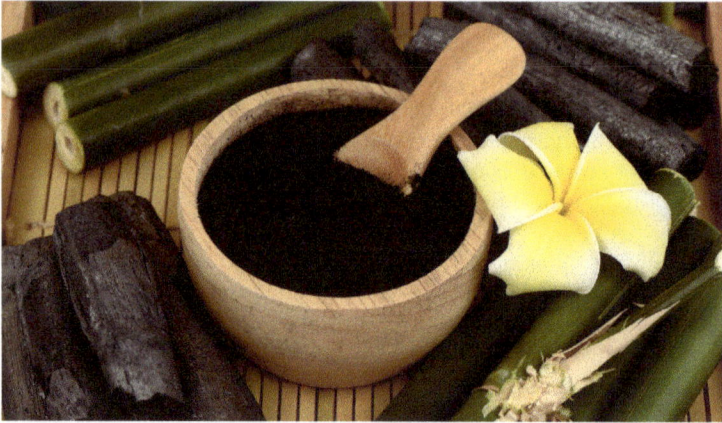

Activated charcoal used as a treatment of aerophagia. shutterstock/wasanajai

Fart, Underwater

It is to be expected that all living creatures that pass gas on land and in the air will do so underwater as well. A large number of humans find this to be a particularly pleasurable activity as confirmed on a large Internet based survey found under the section fart, survey. Of course other animals will release gas underwater as a matter of nature, although they may find it entertaining as well as humans.

 For more information about the sounds generated by underwater farts please see entry on fart, sound (Acoustic, auditory).

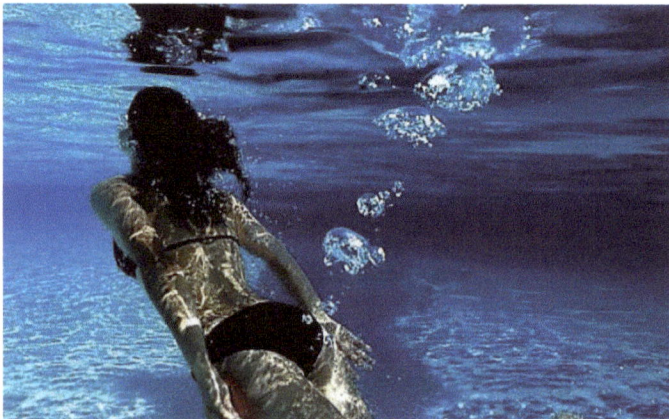

www.home-remedies.br Creative Commons License

The hippopotamus (Greek hippos-horse and potamus-river) is considered by many experts to be the most dangerous animal in Africa (excluding the malaria carrying mosquito) having killed many more people than lions have. The hippo is extremely aggressive with its huge canine teeth and sharp incisors, unpredictable and fearless of humans. Most deaths occur when the victim gets between the hippo and deep water or between a mother and her calf.

Hippos weigh up to 8000 pounds, gallop at 18 M.P.H., sleep or lounge around on riverbanks and in the water most of the day, and graze on the grasslands at night. Their skin secretes sticky pinkish oil that helps protect them from the sun. They defecate generous amounts of excrement into the rivers and ponds in which they wallow all day, punctuated by voluminous farts.

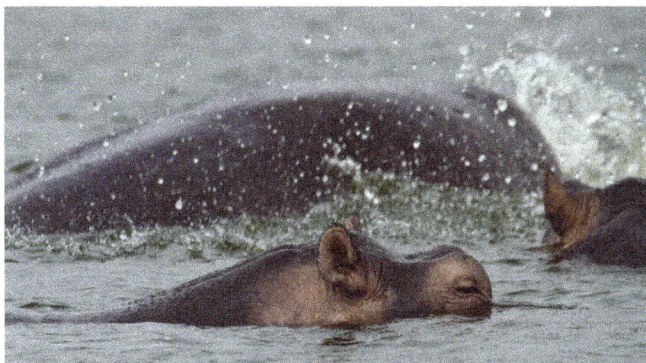

white-voodoo.deviantart.com Creative Commons License

They also participate in marking territory by what the hippo experts refer to as "dung showering." They blow feces mixed with urine over a large area around their watering hole, twirling their relatively short tails like fans to distribute the aromatic spray.

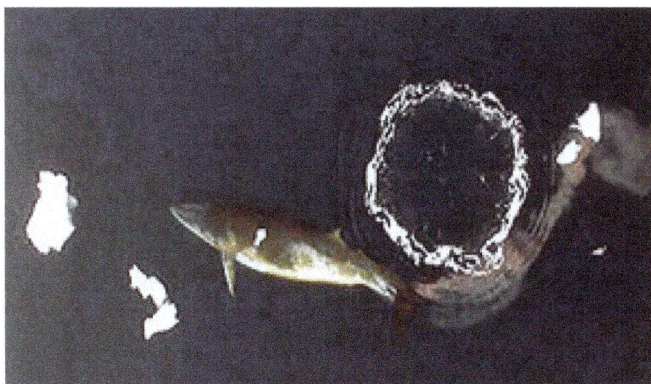

Marine research scientists studying the minke whale population near Antarctica were able to capture a whale fart on film for the first time. The photograph was taken from the bow of the research vessel and the fart subsequently surfaced right under their noses. "We got away from the bow of the ship very quickly ... it does stink," said Nick Gales, a research scientist from the Australian Antarctic Division. However, the skunk like episode did not detract them from completing their mission of collecting DNA from whale dung and attaching satellite tracking devices to the whales to study their migration patterns.

Many fish have a swim bladder that is inflated or deflated as needed to maintain buoyancy. Usually expelled gas exits the mouth but the sand tiger shark, *Carcharias taurus*, discharges it out the anus. The carbon dioxide produced is eliminated via the gills. Methane, hydrogen, and other gasses would typically be released as a fart. Fisherman knew about herring farts and they were even written about back in 1914 by Swedish author Ludvig Runebergwrote in his masterpiece Bottenhavsfiskare (Bothnian Bay Fishermen). The section below is freely translated from the Swedish.

"In the evening they were rowing away to the barren islands, pulled up the boats, lit a fire and made coffee, opened the dinner box and ate. While they were sitting there a group of fishermen were staring out towards the sea, the sun sinking, the sky turning red, and the waves smoothing, wind dying, moon sailing out, lonely and large, the ducks moving back and forth in trains, and in all this, which no longer looked like the earth but more seemed to be an advection into the sky, a distant boiling was seen on the blank water surface. Thousands and thousands of small blisters glaring into the sea, without it being possible to say wherefrom they came, and only in one small defined place: it was the herring which was approaching them on its migration."

Fart, Vagina

Fart is also a term used for an emission or expulsion of air from the vagina. It may occur during or after sexual intercourse or during other sexual acts, stretching, exercise, getting g up from as chair, etcetera. Puffs or small amounts of air passed into the vaginal cavity during cunnilingus are normally not associated with vaginal fart. However "forcing" or purposely blowing air at force into the vaginal cavity can cause an air embolism which is dangerous for the woman, and if pregnant for the fetus.

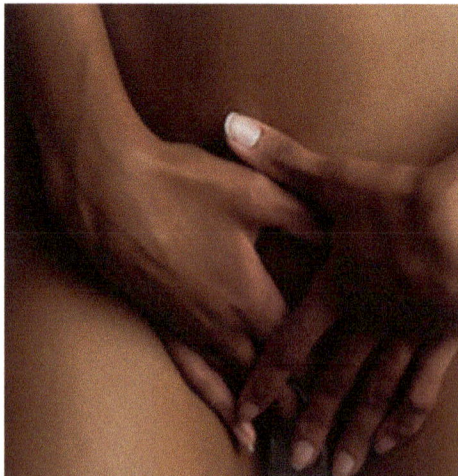

i9.photobucket.com Creative Commons License

The sound of flatus from the vagina is somewhat comparable to flatulence from the anus but does not have a feculent odor in the normal state. If a feculent odor is present it may be because of a colovaginal fistula, a serious condition involving a tear between the vagina and colon. A colovaginal fistula can result from surgery, childbirth, diseases such as the inflammatory bowel disease Crohn disease and other causes. This condition can lead to urinary tract infection and other complications. Slang terms for vaginal flatulence include *vart*, *queef* and *fanny fart*(mostly British).

Fart, Visual

It may sound hard to visualize a fart, but it is actually fairly simple, it's that the circumstances have to be just right. Yes, in releasing an invisible gas into invisible air you would normally not expect to see it with the limited visual spectrum of the human eye. However if you had vision in the infrared portion of the electromagnetic spectrum it would be very visible. With the advent of infrared photography and thermographic imagery the invisible fart can be visualized.

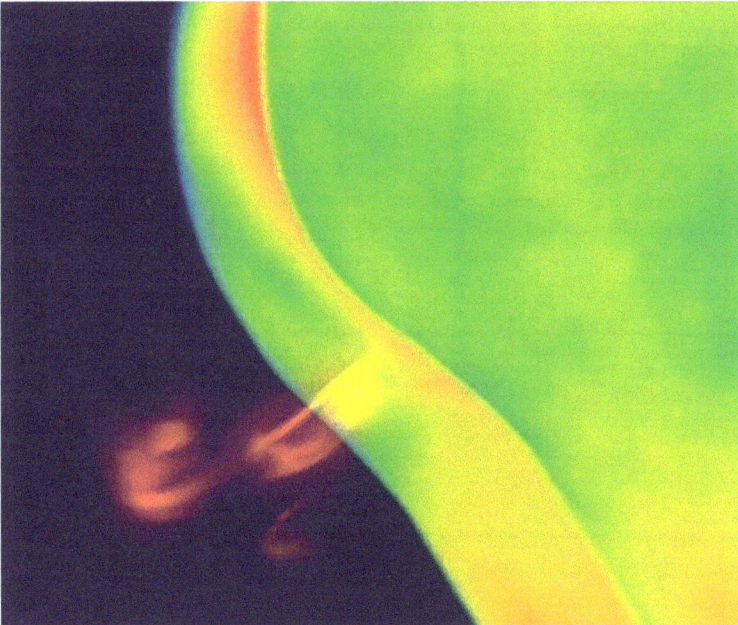

i.telegraph.co.uk

You can also see the fart if the temperature and humidity are just right. If you were in the polar zones, at very high altitude, in frigid weather, or even in a walk-in freezer, dropping a fart from exposed buttocks would look much like the steamy cloud of warm breath on a cold winter day. One should be careful about trying this when it is dangerously frigid as frostbite of this sensitive part of the anatomy may result in a new medical malady, which I hereby name 'frostbutt'.

Frostbite is a real risk for mountaineers, and for Mount Everest climbers the comforts of base camp at an altitude of 17,590 feet may be the last chance they have for a protected bowel movement without exposing their behinds to the extreme winds and weather approaching the summit. Frozen poop stays permanently frozen and does not decompose at that altitude, so there is a growing collection from earlier expeditions that is of concern. Climbers are having a more challenging timed finding ice that has not been contaminated for melting into drinking water. Drinking contaminated water and developing diarrhea would increase the exposure to frostbite dramatically.

The most visible of the visual farts occur in the bathtub or when immersed in water, like a swimming pool or hot whirlpool tub. If you are sharing the water with someone else the innocent looking telltale bubbles underwater, can deliver a powerful bouquet to the unsuspecting nose. The intensity of the olfactory message of the human sense of smell is modulated by the brain and limbic system. If you are in a bathroom having a bowel movement the fart odor is less noticeable and certainly less alarming then when you are in an elevator, theater, or restaurant and you are aromatically assaulted without forewarning.

Fart, Volume (Quantity)

The fact is that all living creatures created gas from the cellular respiration, which is ubiquitous through life forms. The bacteria in your colonic flora generate microscopic nanofarts and microfarts, which collect into larger bubbles of gas in the bowel. They are intermixed with the atmospheric air swallowed throughout the day and particularly at meals, when chewing gum, and chewing or smoking tobacco or other recreational products. Aerophagia is universal and we swallow on average 3-5 cc (teaspoonful) of air with every swallow. Now add into the mixture the gasses produced during the enzymatic digestive processes as well as the neutralization of gastric hydrochloric acid and pancreatic and duodenal bicarbonate and you have a virtual windstorm of voluminous gasses transiting the bowel.

Fortunately the vast majority of the gasses produced are absorbed by the gut, then into the bloodstream through diffusion and as a solution, finally being exhaled when they reach the alveoli of the lungs and can be exchanged with atmospheric air. The component gasses have very different properties of diffusion through the vowel wall and into the bloodstream. Carbon dioxide readily diffuses and enters solution and is exhaled, such that although it is the largest volume of gas generated by far, and temporarily is a major contributor to distension and postprandial (after meal) discomfort, it is the easiest to eliminate from the bowel and is only a minor contributor to flatulence.

Nitrogen is the largest volume component of atmospheric air, and as would be expected, represents an identically high proportion of the gasses swallowed through aerophagia. Once in the body the carbon dioxide of the air is absorbed and eliminated as discussed above. The nitrogen however is a very poorly absorbed gas, and in essence will either come back up as a burp, or will sooner or later, comes out the other end as a fart.

The oxygen in the air, representing nearly 21% of the air gasses swallowed during aerophagia, is absorbed slowly, as the gut is not nearly as efficient as the lungs for respiration. As the carbon dioxide and oxygen are absorbed the percent of the gastrointestinal tract air that is nitrogen increases. As soon as the digestive process begins, hydrochloric acid of the stomach is neutralized by bicarbonate of the duodenum and pancreas. Large volumes of carbon dioxide gas are generated, as are smaller quantities of hydrogen, methane and other aromatic gasses discussed later. The volume of gasses in the gastrointestinal tract is dependent on the quantity and nature if foods ingested, the body's ability to synthesize and utilize specific enzymes for the various food types, the nature and quantity of the bacteria in the gut flora, the speed of gastrointestinal transit which may be influences by drugs, hormones, food product and illness, the absorptive capacity and health of the mucosal lining, and the physical length of the individuals gastrointestinal tract.

The question of what is the average number of farts per day is similar to the question if what is an average price for a normal used car. What year, make, model, condition, diesel or gas or electric or hybrid, mileage, etc. etc. The quoted figure of 11.5 farts per day is a reasonable approximation from a very small sample size of male medical students, but normal has a very wide range depending on the variables. The female medical students were too smart to participate in the study so a far as science is concerned, women do not fart. Later suggestions that they fart, but less than the guys, is just as suspect.
The differences in the physical attributes between male and female of a species represent their sexual dimorphism. The theory of sexual selection advanced by Charles Darwin in 1871 is closely related to sexual dimorphism. On average adult humans males are on 4% taller and 8% heavier than females. In a number of other species it is the female that is larger, occasionally dramatically so.

The triple wart sea devil, an anglerfish, exhibits extreme sexual dimorphism, with the male becoming little more than a stunted sperm-producing body that lives a parasitic existence off of the females hard work and effort in providing livelihood and producing the next generation of offspring. Some human males appear to have evolved their behavioral patterns from the anglerfish modus operandi.
In most mammals, humans included, the males are larger in size, mass, and caloric intake. In most species is the make that is diminutive in size, sometimes dramatically so. It would only make sense that makes would generate more gas, but how do the two compare if the caloric intake and composition were identical. Since there are no identically comparable cases studies would have to be average large populations of each gender and minimize the variables as much as possible.

As curious as we may be to know the answer to this question vital to gender politics and security, no studies are planned or anticipated. There have been reports of extreme flatulence in the medical literature of what may be considered the upper limits of the normal range, up to 150 in a 24-hour period. There are probably more accurate reports of what is the upper limit of spousal tolerance in divorce court proceedings and depositions. So for general health we talk about achieving our target heart rate during exercise. Is there an equivalent for a target fart rate? For harmonious relationships ideal would be below the quoted figure of 11.5 farts per day, that way you could reasonably attest that you fart less than average. You could also argue that the 23 you passed were each only half fart so you still are within the normal range.

As we age we produce less digestive enzymes and there is an argument to be made that there should be an adjustment and tolerance allowed for 'old farts'. The sheer number of variables allow 101 + explanations for why you fart much less than expected for your given circumstances. But perhaps the best excuse is that you did not do anything, it's the billions of nanofarting and microfarting bacteria that are to blame. If you are told to pick on someone closer to your own size you could blame the dog and claim it is a talented ventrilo-farter. Trying to arrive at a definition of what constitutes a discrete individual fart is a challenge worthy of drafting and approving a United Nations resolution. Is a staccato stutter often small farts completed in rapid succession to count as 1 or ten? Is one large long loud fart the equivalent of four small farts over 30 seconds. Should a loud tuba blast count the same as a faint toot?

Fart, Weight

As a fart is composed of atoms and molecules it has physical properties, including a mass and weight. Since it is composed of gasses and volatile molecules it is very light, yet the weight is measureable. Each fart is unique, much like fingerprints, although don't expect it to be used for personal identification. The total mass of the average fart is 0.0371 grams. For those wishing to lose weight every fart means you weigh just a little bit less. The constituent gasses and mass of the average fart is listed below:

Nitrogen: 0.0263 grams
Hydrogen: 0.0003 grams
Carbon Dioxide: 0.0063 grams
Methane: 0.0018 grams
Oxygen: 0.0016 grams
Odiferous Products: 0.0008 grams

Fiber

Dietary fiber, also referred to as roughage is the indigestible component of plants consumed as food. There are two main types, differentiated by their solubility in water. Soluble fiber, which dissolves in water, is readily fermented in the intestinal tract producing gases and byproducts. It us further divided into viscous fiber and prebiotic fiber. Is commonly found in oat bran, beans, peas, and most fruits.

Insoluble fiber does not dissolve in water. It is further divided into fiber that is metabolically inert and simply provides added bulk and fluid retention, or prebiotic which is metabolically fermented by the gut flora. The bulk enhancing fibers ease defecation both by adding moisture to the stool as well as stimulating gut peristalsis and colonic mass movements.

The added bulk also reduces the incidence of spasmodic contractions of the bowel, which may contribute to the pain, and discomfort of irritable bowel syndrome, previously known as a spastic colon or spastic colitis. This is the type of fiber found in wheat bran and some vegetables. Dietary fiber is comprised of non-starch polysaccharides such as arabinoxylans, cellulose, resistant starch, resistant dextrins, inulin, lignin, waxes, chitins, pectins, beta-glucans, and oligosaccharides.

Lignin, a major dietary insoluble fiber source, may alter the rate and metabolism of soluble fibers. Lignin is found in high concentrations in tree bark and its difficulty in being digested and decomposed played a major role in the Carboniferous era when tree bark was a multiple of the thickness it is today. On the other hand, insoluble fibers like the resistant starches are fully fermented. The main disadvantage of a diet high in fiber is the increased intestinal gas production with bloating and being a social outcast as a possible consequence.

Soluble fiber can be found in foods such as oatbran, barley, nuts, seeds, beans, lentils, fruits (citrus, apples), strawberries and many vegetables

Insoluble fiber is found in foods such as whole wheat and whole grain products, vegetables, and wheat bran

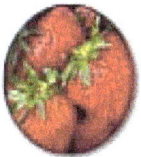

Soluble fiber sources

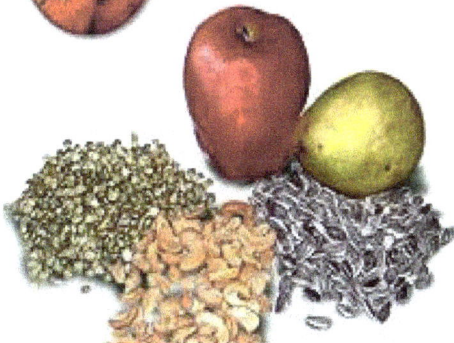

Insoluble fiber sources

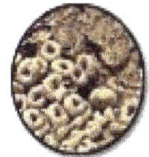

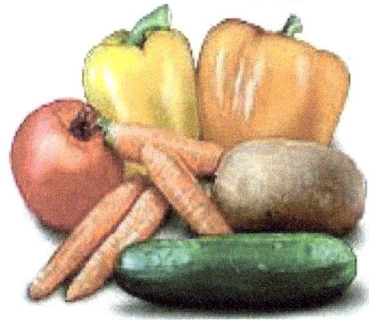

The original definition of fiber was the components of plants that were not affected by digestive enzymes, a definition that includes lignin and

polysaccharides. The definition was later expanded to include resistant starches, polysaccharides, lignin, and inulin with other oligosaccharides. While dietary fiber is present in nearly all fruits and vegetables, the type and quantity of fiber varies widely. Persimmons have safety issues and if eaten unripen the soluble tannin shiboul can lead to gastric phytobezoars a condition where a hardened wood like mass of fiber remains within the stomach for years or a lifetime.

Soluble fiber is present, in variable quantities, in plant food including legumes (peas, soybeans, lupins, beans), oats, rye, chia, and barley, some fruits and fruit juices (including prune juice, plums, berries, ripe bananas, apples, and pears), certain vegetables such as broccoli, carrots, Jerusalem artichokes, root tubers and root vegetables such as sweet potatoes and onions (skins of these are sources of insoluble fiber also), psyllium seed husk (a mucilage soluble fiber) and flax seeds, and nuts, with almonds being the highest in dietary fiber

Fiber Content Of Popular Foods			
Food Source	Soluble Fiber (g)	Insoluble Fiber (g)	Total Fiber (g)
Apple (1 med)	0.9g	2.0g	2.9g
Banana (1 med)	0.6g	1.4g	2.0g
Orange (1 med)	1.3g	0.7g	2.0g
Broccoli (1 stalk)	1.3g	1.4g	2.7g
Carrots (1 large)	1.3g	1.6g	2.9g
Tomato (1 small)	0.1g	0.7g	0.8g
Potato (1 medium)	1.0g	0.8g	1.8g
All Bran (1/2 cup)	1.4g	7.6g	9.0g
Oat Bran (1/2 cup)	2.2g	2.2g	4.4g
Corn Flakes (1 cup)	0g	0.5g	0.5g
Rolled Oats (3/4 cup)	1.3g	1.7g	3.0g
Wheat Bread (1 slice)	0.3g	1.1g	1.4g
White Bread (1 slice)	0.3g	0.1g	0.4g
Green Peas (2/3 cup)	0.6g	3.3g	3.9g
Kidney Beans (1/2 cup)	1.6g	4.9g	6.5g
Lentils (2/3 cup)	0.6g	3.9g	4.5g

source: USDA/ARS Nutrient Data Laboratory

Public Domain

Sources of insoluble fiber include, whole grain foods, wheat and corn bran, legumes such as beans and peas, nuts and seeds, potato skins, lignins, vegetables such as green beans, cauliflower, zucchini (courgette), celery, nopal, some fruits including avocado, and unripe bananas, the skins of some fruits, including kiwifruit, grapes and tomatoes. Vegetable gum fiber, such as guar gum and acacia Senegal gum, dissolve easily and have no aftertaste making them a popular fiber supplement additive.

Dietary fibers have three primary mechanisms: bulking, viscosity and fermentation. As they can change the nature and transit of the intestinal contents they may impact how other nutrients and materials are absorbed. Some soluble fibers bind to bile acids preventing their normal reabsorption in the small intestine this interruption in the normal enterohepatic circulation of the bile from the small intestine to the liver results in the loss of cholesterol in the form of bile acids via the stool. The cholesterol levels in the blood are subsequently lowered since the liver removes cholesterol from the circulation to synthesize replacement bile salts. Viscous soluble fibers may also inhibit the absorption of sugar thus reducing the sugar insulin response after meals.

Fatty foods and hypertonic solutions delay gastric emptying and gut transit time. The intestinal contents are called chyme once they leave the stomach. Chyme consists of food compounds, digestive enzymes, stomach acid and pancreatic and duodenal bicarbonate, bile acids, complex lipids in changing micellar, aqueous, hydrocolloid, hydrophobic, and hydrophilic phases all in a mixture of solid, liquid, colloidal and gas bubble phases. In other words, it is one chaotic churning, digesting, fermenting mass with selectively absorbs ion and secretion occurring throughout the process. Non-absorbed carbohydrates such as pectin, gum Arabic, oligosaccharides and resistant starch, are fermented by the gut flora to short-chain fatty acids (mainly acetic, propionic and n-butyric), carbon dioxide, hydrogen and methane. The colon will absorb nearly all of the short-chain fatty acids with the butyric acid being utilized as the main source of energy for colonic cells.

Soluble and insoluble fiber both increases food volume without additional caloric content. The increased volume can provide greater satiety, which may eat to decreased food intake and weight loss. Intestinal fermentation can increase the production of beneficial short chain fatty acids. Soluble fiber absorbs water and forms a viscous gel, known as a hydrophilic mucelloid that slows gastric emptying and intestinal transit. The increase bulk may shield carbohydrates from enzymes, delay the absorption of glucose, and reduce the fluctuations of blood sugar levels that result. On the other and the delayed transit allows more time for enzymatic activity as well as fermentation by the gut flora.

Insoluble fiber enhances gut motility and speeds transit time, as well as adding bulk and moisture to the stool promoting defecation and preventing constipation. Current recommendations for daily dietary fiber intake are 30 grams for the average adults. The average American consumes about half of that amount. Sugars and starches provide 4 Calories per gram as the digestive system has enzymes to break them down into the simple absorbable sugars of glucose, fructose, and galactose. Insoluble fiber cannot be digested so no calories are absorbed. Soluble fiber is partially fermented, and the caloric intake is determined by the degree that it is broken down into absorbable nutrients. As a result of the variability in calories generated there is controversy on their calorie count. 2 Calories per gram of soluble fiber is a reasonable compromise. Fibers with partial or low ferment ability include cellulose, hemicellulose, lignans, plant waxes, and resistant starches. Fibers with high ferment ability include beta-glucans, pectins, natural gums, inulins, oligosaccharides, and resistant dextrins.

Flatology

The scientific study of flatulence is termed flatology. Flatulence is defined as flatus (Latin blowing) expelled through the anus as well as the state of being affected with gases in the intestinal tract. The noises commonly associated with flatulence ("Blowing a raspberry") are caused by the vibration of the anal sphincter and occasionally by the buttocks. Both the noise and smell associated with flatus leaving the anus can be sources of embarrassment or comedy in many cultures. There are five general symptoms related to intestinal gas: pain, bloating and abdominal distension, excessive flatus volume, excessive flatus smell and gas incontinence.

Flatulence

Flatulence is defined as flatus (Latin blowing) expelled through the anus as well as the state of being affected with gases in the intestinal tract. The scientific study of flatulence is termed flatology .The noises commonly associated with flatulence are caused by the vibration of the anal sphincter and occasionally by the buttocks. Both the noise and smell associated with flatus leaving the anus can be sources of embarrassment or comedy in many cultures. Further characterizations of the nature of flatulence are found under the topics of fart, flatus, and intestinal gas, which are commonly used, interchangeably in the English language.

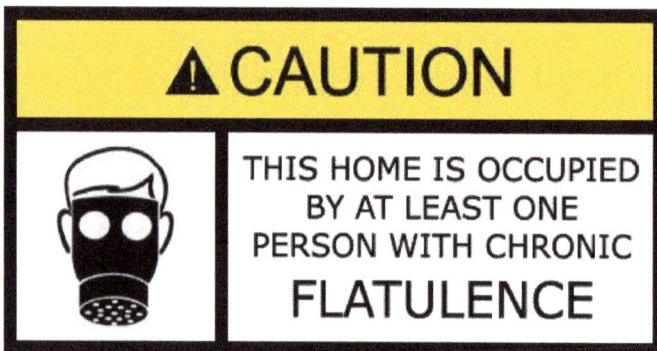

⚠ CAUTION

THIS HOME IS OCCUPIED BY AT LEAST ONE PERSON WITH CHRONIC FLATULENCE

unclestinky.files.wordpress.com Creative Commons License

FODMAP Diet

FODMAP is an acronym that stands for Fermentable Oligosaccharides, Disaccharides, Monosaccharides, And Polyols. These short chain carbohydrates and related sugar alcohols are poorly absorbed in the small intestine.. Many of the sugar alcohols including sorbitol, mannitol, xylitol, isomalt, and maltitol are added to commercial food products as non-nutritive bulk sweeteners. Originally developed at Monash University in Melbourne, Australia it has become popular worldwide as a means of reducing the symptoms of irritable bowel syndrome, functional gastrointestinal disorders, and excess intestinal gas

Foods suitable on a low-fodmap diet

fruit	vegetables	grain foods	milk products	other
fruit banana, blueberry, boysenberry, canteloupe, cranberry, durian, grape, grapefruit, honeydew melon, kiwifruit, lemon, lime, mandarin, orange, passionfruit, pawpaw, raspberry, rhubarb, rockmelon, star anise, strawberry, tangelo Note: if fruit is dried, eat in small quantities	**vegetables** alfalfa, artichoke, bamboo shoots, bean shoots, bok choy, carrot, celery, choko, choy sum, endive, ginger, green beans, lettuce, olives, parsnip, potato, pumpkin, red capsicum (bell pepper), silver beet, spinach, summer squash (yellow), swede, sweet potato, taro, tomato, turnip, yam, zucchini **herbs** basil, chili, coriander, ginger, lemongrass, marjoram, mint, oregano, parsley, rosemary, thyme	**cereals** gluten-free bread or cereal products **bread** 100% spelt bread **rice** **oats** **polenta** **other** arrowroot, millet, psyllium, quinoa, sorgum, tapioca	**milk** lactose-free milk, oat milk*, rice milk, soy milk* *check for additives **cheeses** hard cheeses, and brie and camembert **yoghurt** lactose-free varieties **ice-cream substitutes** gelati, sorbet **butter substitutes** olive oil	**sweeteners** sugar* (sucrose), glucose, artificial sweeteners not ending in '-ol' **honey substitutes** golden syrup*, maple syrup*, molasses, treacle *small quantities

3.bp.blogspot.com Creative Commons License

Eliminate foods containing fodmaps

excess fructose	lactose	fructans	galactans	polyols
fruit apple, mango, nashi, pear, tinned fruit in natural juice, watermelon **sweeteners** fructose, high fructose corn syrup **large total fructose dose** concentrated fruit sources, large serves of fruit, dried fruit, fruit juice **honey** corn syrup, fruisana	**milk** milk from cows, goats or sheep, custard, ice cream, yoghurt **cheeses** soft unripened cheeses eg. cottage, cream, mascarpone, ricotta	**vegetables** asparagus, beetroot, broccoli, brussels sprouts, cabbage, eggplant, fennel, garlic, leek, okra, onion (all), shallots, spring onion **cereals** wheat and rye, in large amounts eg. bread, crackers, cookies, couscous, pasta **fruit** custard apple, persimmon, watermelon **miscellaneous** chicory, dandelion, inulin	**legumes** baked beans, chickpeas, kidney beans, lentils	**fruit** apple, apricot, avocado, blackberry, cherry, lychee, nashi, nectarine, peach, pear, plum, prune, watermelon **vegetables** cauliflower, green capsicum (bell pepper), mushroom, sweet corn **sweeteners** sorbitol (420) mannitol (421) isomalt (953) maltitol (965) xylitol (967)

bp.blogspot.com Creative Commons License

Food Intolerance

Food intolerance is often very individualized and is not the same as food allergy. In food allergy the food that triggers the reaction is known as the antigen, and the allergic reaction is mediated by the body's immune and inflammatory response systems. The chart following identifies several of the other differences.

Allergy	Intolerance
Obvious symptoms	Subtle symptoms
Immediate reaction - within one hour	Delayed reaction - 12 to 72 hours
Rapid onset of symptoms and often reaction magnifies with each exposure	Slow onset and often slow magnification of symptoms, even after the often long delay
Often triggered by minute amount of food	Not predominantly affected by food quantity
Affects Immunoglobulin E (IgE)	Affects Immunoglobulin G (IgG) and/or other mechanisms (prostaglandins, leukotrienes, etc.)
Allergies are uncommon	Intolerances are very common
Generally non-reversible	Reversible
Well recognised by medicine	Just beginning to be recognised by medicine
Test : Prick or RAST (Radio-immunodiffusion Test)	Test : Electro-Dermal Screening (EDS) or Blood Immunoglobulin G (IgG)

lunar.thegamez.net Creative Commons License

 In a number of cases of food intolerance the sensitivity is the result of lower levels of the necessary enzymes to digest specific foods. For example the milk sugar lactose requires the specific enzyme called lactase, to properly digest this complex sugar into absorbable simple sugars. If insufficient lactase is present the gut flora, which is comprised of various microorganisms, ferments the residual undigested sugar. This process leads to the release of various gases that may accumulate within the digestive tract and are eliminated as a fart. A portion of the gas is produced such as carbon dioxide are readily absorbed by the digestive tract and transported by the circulatory system to the lungs where they are eliminated through respiration.

The ability of the individual to produce the necessary lactase enzyme is often hereditary. Many populations have limited lactase production, which results in the common occurrence of lactose intolerance. If the intake of lactose is restricted the limited amount of lactase president may be sufficient to prevent the development of the symptoms of lactose intolerance. These symptoms such as excess intestinal gas diarrhea abdominal cramps are often dependent on the quantity of lactose ingested that exceeds the available lactase enzyme necessary for its digestion.

A number of the digestive enzymes, which are lacking in individual populations, can be supplemented either by purchased enzyme products, or by the production of the enzymes by the individuals gut flora. The flora may be supplemented with commensal organisms such as lactobacillus, which aid in the digestion of dairy products. Other commonly malabsorbed complex sugars include fructose, mannitol, sorbitol, and a variety of sugar substitutes.

Food Intolerance and Common Symptoms

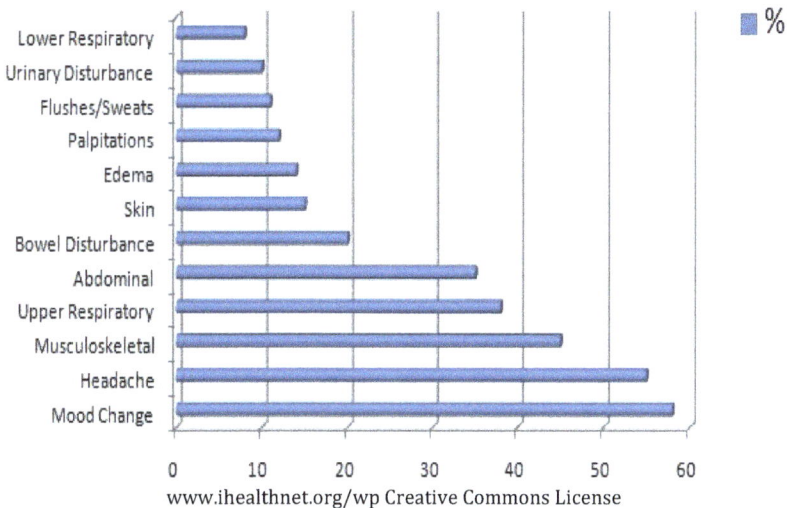

www.ihealthnet.org/wp Creative Commons License

Fructose in particular has limited enzyme available for its digestion and frequently leads to intolerance when ingested beyond the enzyme capacity. In some cases the necessary enzyme for digestion of the complex sugar or starch does not naturally occur in humans. One example is the enzyme cellulase, which is required for the digestion of cellulose a sugar commonly found in plants. This enzyme is found in herbivorous animals that consume grasses and cellulose containing food products.

The complex sugars found in legumes are in the raffinose class, which includes Stachyose and Verbascose. The enzyme required for their digestion is called Alpha galactosidase. This enzyme is not naturally occurring in humans and must be obtained from external sources. Without the availability of this enzyme the gut flora metabolism releases large quantities of gases, which are often released as a fart. The enzyme is found naturally in beans and legumes once the seed is germinated. The enzyme is also available commercially as over-the-counter products such as Beano, Say Yes to Beans, and other products.

Many individuals also have difficulty digesting the cereal grains, especially those that contain gluten. Gluten intolerance may range from mild excess gaseous us to true inflammation and damage of the intestinal lining. When the villi, which are the fingerlike projections of the bowel lining, are damaged malabsorption occurs. This condition known as gluten sensitive enteropathy (also known as celiac disease and celiac sprue) is a serious health concern. Adherence to a strict gluten-free diet is required to prevent further injury and complications from the malabsorption of nutrients and other features of the disorder.

A number of the food in tolerances may be addressed easily by avoiding the inciting foods in the diet. A number of food in tolerances are more challenging to control by diet alone as the commercial food products in the marketplace may contain small quantities. It is necessary to carefully read the ingredients of all commercial food products purchased or consumed if one has specific food intolerance. With further understanding of the gut microbiome, Pre-biotics and probiotics maybe used to have commensals microbes supplement the natural enzymes of the human host. There are a wide variety of food intolerances and enzyme deficiencies and that can be major contributors to gastrointestinal and other symptoms. Enzymes deficiencies are not uncommon and there are many possible enzymes to investigate including proteases such as pepsin, pepsinogen, trypsin, trypsinogen, chymotrypsin, and chymotrypsinogen. Other enzymes include amylase, lipase, invertase, sucrose, maltase, lactase, and about 1,600 others.

Taking a Sherlock Holmes approach and trying an elimination diet is certainly reasonable. Enzyme supplements are commercially available and are another approach for an empiric trial if the suspect foods are not well defined. It is important to take the appropriate enzyme with the appropriate food. The right enzyme for the wrong food, or the wrong enzyme for the right food, will not make a bit of difference in helping your digestion. The most common enzyme deficiency is lactase resulting in lactose intolerance. Medications can also interfere with enzyme activity and give rise to digestive symptoms

The most widely distributed naturally occurring non-enzyme food chemical capable of provoking reactions is salicylate, with tartrazine and benzoic acid sensitivity seen less often. Benzoates and salicylates occur naturally in many different foods, including fruits, juices, vegetables, tomatoes, spices, herbs, nuts, tea, wines, and coffee. Other natural chemicals, which commonly cause reactions and cross reactivity, include amines, nitrates, sulphites and some antioxidants. Reactions to chocolate, cheese, bananas, avocado, tomato or wine suggest that bioactive amines may be a likely candidate as a food chemical that triggers sensitivities.

Franklin, Benjamin

Benjamin Franklin (1706-1790) was a polymath scientist, author, statesman, philosopher, publisher, diplomat, inventor, and humorist. In 1781 he was serving as the United States ambassador to France and with his scientific background kept in close communication with the European community of scientists. As is typical for a scientific congress an announcement from the Royal Academy of Brussels was made calling for the presentation of scientific papers on a host of subjects.

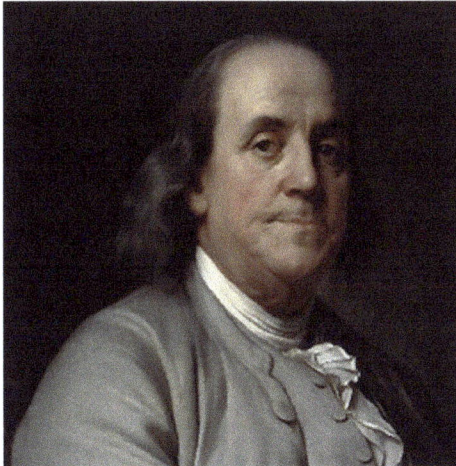

Portrait of Benjamin Franklin by Joseph Siffrein Duplessis c. 1785 National Portrait Gallery Washington D.C. Public Domain

Franklin found some of the proposals so pretentious that his "bawdy, scurrilous nature" was stirred to compose a satirical response in the form of a proposal for research. As an illustrious statesman and scientist his proposal would demand serious attention. His proposal to the Royal Academy of Brussels is reprinted in its entirety in the companion volume to this book *Artsy Fartsy, Cultural History of the Fart*.

"Let every fart count as a peal of thunder for liberty. Let every fart remind the nation of how much it has let pass out of its control. So fart, and if you must, fart often. But always fart without apology. Fart for freedom, fart for liberty… and fart proudly!"

"He that lives upon Hope, dies farting." is another of his famous quotes.

His proposal to the Royal Academy (reprinted in full below) called for scientific research to discover food additives that would provide a variety of attractive aromas to produce good smelling farts that would be socially welcomed.

Fructose

Fructose, fruit sugar, is a simple monosaccharide found in many fruits, berries, flowers, honey, artichokes, wheat, onions, and root vegetables. Fructose was discovered in 1847 by the French chemist Augustin-Pierre Dubrunfaut. It is prepared commercially from sugar cane, sugar beets, and corn. High-fructose corn syrup (HFCS) is made from the enzymatic conversion of cornstarch and is often added as a sweetener to soft drinks and other foods.

Apples and pears contain more than twice as much free fructose as glucose. High concentrations of free fructose in these fruits and their juices can cause diarrhea in children, as they are unable to absorb fructose as well as glucose and sucrose. The fructose creates higher osmolality in the small intestine drawing water into the gastrointestinal tract resulting in diarrhea. It is because of the fructose that apple juice; raisins, grape juice, and bananas will increase flatulence.

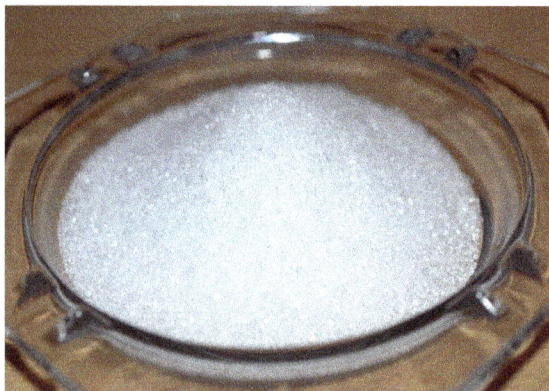

Crystalline fructose Creative Commons License

Fructose exists in foods either as a monosaccharide (free fructose) or as a unit of a disaccharide (sucrose). Fructose is seventy-three percent sweeter than sucrose. The enzyme sucrase catalyzes sucrose into glucose and fructose, both of which are absorbed by the small intestine, as is the other monosaccharide galactose. Fructose has a very low glycemic index of nineteen, compared with one hundred for glucose and sixty-eight for sucrose.

Fructose Intolerance, Hereditary

Dietary fructose intolerance is the decreased capacity to absorb fructose because of deficient fructose carriers in the small intestine's enterocytes. Hereditary fructose intolerance is a more serious liver enzyme deficiency that requires total abstinence from fructose. Hereditary fructose intolerance is a defect of fructose metabolism caused by an autosomal recessive gene mutation resulting in a deficiency of the enzyme aldolase B. Hereditary fructose intolerance individuals are asymptomatic until they ingest fructose, sucrose, or sorbitol. Symptoms can include vomiting, hypoglycemia, jaundice, hemorrhage, hepatomegaly, hyperuricemia and kidney failure.

The pathways of fructose in HFI & Fructose Malabsorption

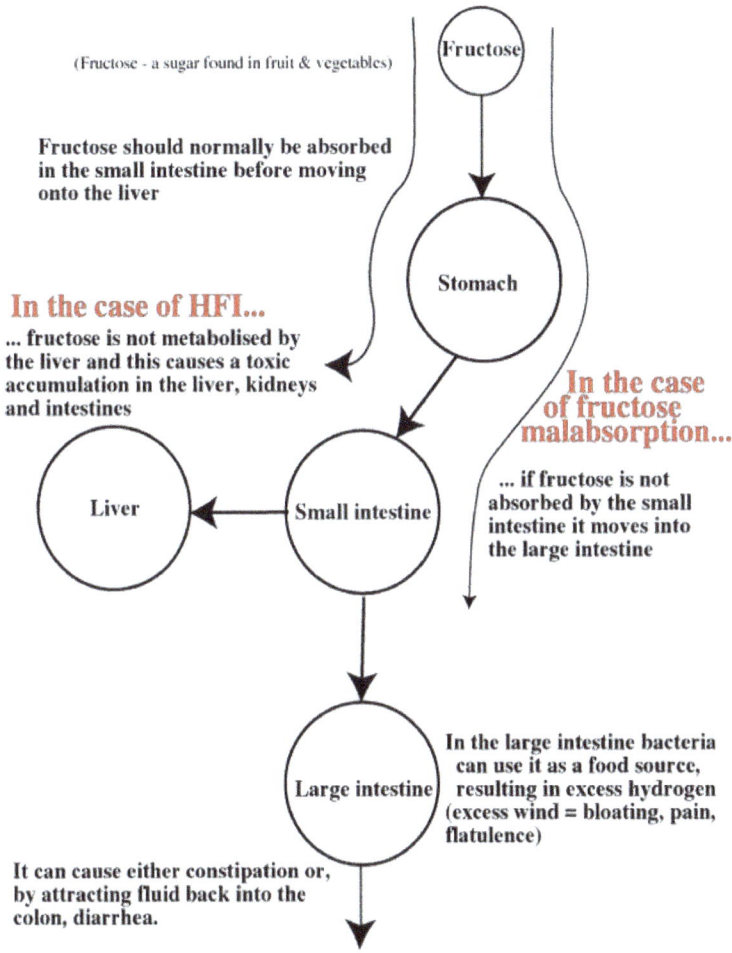

(Fructose - a sugar found in fruit & vegetables)

Fructose

Fructose should normally be absorbed in the small intestine before moving onto the liver

Stomach

In the case of HFI...

... fructose is not metabolised by the liver and this causes a toxic accumulation in the liver, kidneys and intestines

In the case of fructose malabsorption...

... if fructose is not absorbed by the small intestine it moves into the large intestine

Liver

Small intestine

Large intestine

In the large intestine bacteria can use it as a food source, resulting in excess hydrogen (excess wind = bloating, pain, flatulence)

It can cause either constipation or, by attracting fluid back into the colon, diarrhea.

Creative Commons License

Diagnosis of hereditary fructose intolerance is suspected in infants who become symptomatic when fructose-containing foods are introduced into their diet. Affected individuals are asymptomatic and healthy, provided they do not ingest foods containing fructose or its precursors sucrose and sorbitol.

Fructose is absorbed in the small intestine without the need for digestive enzymes. About 25–50 grams of fructose per intake can be properly absorbed in healthy people. People with fructose malabsorption cannot absorb more than 25 grams per intake. In the large intestine the fructose is metabolized into short chain fatty acids, producing hydrogen, carbon dioxide and methane. The increased osmotic load can cause diarrhea. The abnormal increase in hydrogen is detectable with the hydrogen breath test.

Foods that contain more glucose than fructose are usually well tolerated since glucose enhances absorption of fructose. Foods with a high fructose to glucose ratio like apples and pears can be difficult to process and sound are avoided. Additional foods to be avoided include those rich in fructans such as artichokes, asparagus, leeks, onions, wheat, sorbitol, xylitol, erythritol, inulin, fructo-oligosaccharide, and mannitol.

Fructose Malabsorption

Fructose malabsorption, formerly named hereditary fructose intolerance or dietary fructose intolerance, is the decreased capacity to absorb fructose because of deficient fructose carriers in the small intestine's enterocytes. This condition is common in patients with irritable bowel syndrome. It is not synonymous with the more serious hereditary fructose intolerance, a liver enzyme deficiency that requires total abstinence from fructose.

How Much Fructose Can I Eat Per Day?

We can only absorb 20 grams of Fructose per day. That's 4 ½ teaspoons or two apples.

Any more is harmful to the liver, causing fat deposits, obesity, and insulin resistance.

Fructose in fresh fruit

Fruit portion	Grams of Fructose
1 lime	0.0
1 lemon	0.6
1 cup cranberries	0.7
1 date	2.6
1/8 cantaloupe	2.8
1 cup raspberries	3.0
1 kiwi	3.4
1 slice pineapple	4.0
1 grapefruit	4.3
1 tangerine	4.8
1 peach/nectarine	5.8
1 orange	6.1
1/2 papaya	6.3
1 banana	7.1
1 cup blueberries	7.4
1 apple	9.5
1 pear	11.8
¾ cup raisins	12.3
1 cup grapes	12.4
1/2 mango	16.2
1 cup dry apricots	16.4
1 cup dry figs	23.0

Creative Commons License

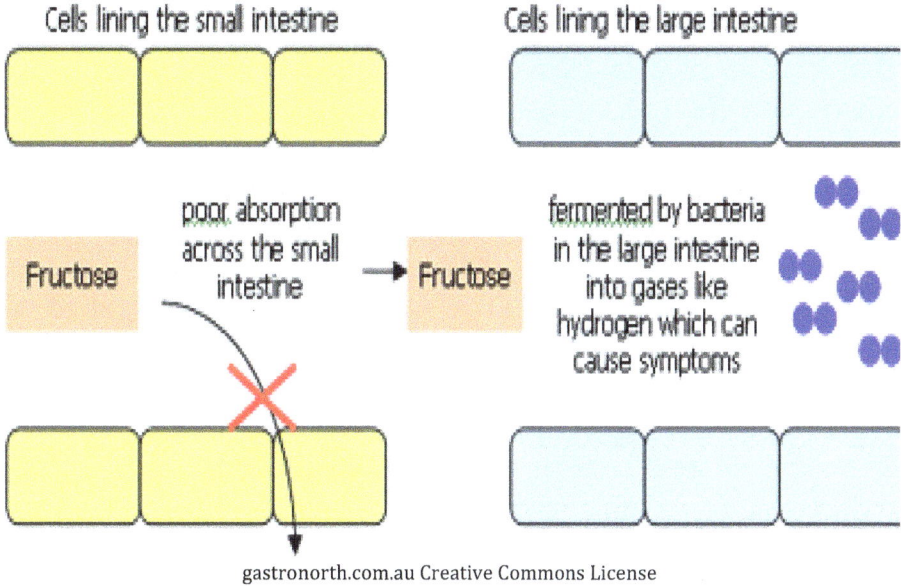

Cells lining the small intestine

Cells lining the large intestine

Fructose

poor absorption across the small intestine →

Fructose

fermented by bacteria in the large intestine into gases like hydrogen which can cause symptoms

gastronorth.com.au Creative Commons License

Gas, Therapy (see Intestinal Gas Therapy)

Gastroesophageal Reflux Disease (GERD)

Gastroesophageal reflux disease (GERD) is mucosal damage of the esophagus caused by the reflux of gastric acid, bile, and digestive enzymes. In Western populations GERD affects approximately ten to twenty percent of the population. The most common symptom is heartburn, formally known as pyrosis. In the United States twenty percent of people have symptoms in a given week, and seven percent every day.

GERD is usually caused by abnormal relaxation of the lower esophageal sphincter or hiatal hernia with contributing factors such as obesity, Zollinger-Ellison hypergastrinemia, hypercalcemia, scleroderma, and esophageal dysmotility. Carminatives, drugs, hormones, alcohol, tobacco, fried or fatty foods, and chocolate all of which can reduce the lower esophageal sphincter pressure can aggravate it.

Treatment is typically via lifestyle changes and medications such as proton pump inhibitors, H2 receptor blockers or antacids. Some Antacids can be absorbed leading to an alkalosis syndrome. Antacids also generate large volumes of carbon dioxide as they neutralize the gastric hydrochloric acid, Magnesium containing antacids can cause diarrhea, aluminum containing antacids can cause constipation, and often a combination of the two is used to minimize the impact on bowel movements, Calcium based antacids can lead to a rebound of acid secretion is calcium is a stimulant of gastric acid production.

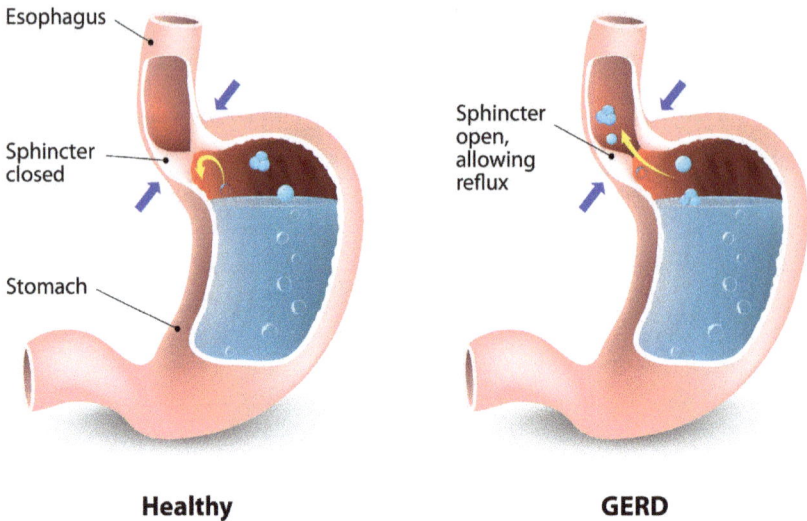

Esophagus

Sphincter closed

Stomach

Sphincter open, allowing reflux

Healthy   **GERD**

Gastroesophageal Reflux Disease shutterstock/designua

Surgery treatment with tightening of the lower esophageal sphincter has a similar response rate as medications. If inadequately treated GERD may progress to Barrett's esophagus with intestinal metaplasia where the epithelial cells transition from the normal esophageal squamous epithelium to intestinal columnar epithelium. With the development of atypia and dysplasia this can progress to the development of adenocarcinoma of the esophagus. If Barrett's esophagus has developed a screening endoscopy with biopsies to evaluate for dysplasia is suggested.

The diagnosis of GERD is usually by history with typical symptoms of heartburn and reflux. Atypical manifestations of GERD include laryngitis, unexplained chest pain, chronic cough, sinusitis, pulmonary fibrosis, earache, recurrent ear infections, asthma, and obstructive sleep apnea. Another unusual symptom is called water brash, which is a rush of salivary secretions after an episode of regurgitation to dilute and clear the acid in the esophagus.

A possible cardiac cause of atypical chest should be excluded before ascribing the source to GERD. Approximately 40% of GERD patients have a Helicobacter pylori infection. The eradication of Helicobacter pylori can lead to a worsening of the GERD symptoms since the resolving gastritis leads to an increase in gastric acid secretion.

The current gold standard for diagnosis of GERD is esophageal pH monitoring. Endoscopy is advised if any alarm symptoms are present including dysphagia, anemia, and blood in the stool, wheezing, weight loss, respiratory or laryngeal symptoms. Long-standing or severe symptoms would also prompt endoscopic evaluation for   Barrett's esophagus and dysplasia.

The treatments for GERD include lifestyle modifications, medications, and possibly surgery. Initial treatment is typically with a proton-pump inhibitor or histamine 2 blocker that usually provides prompt and significant relief. Weight loss, avoiding large heavy meals, not lying down, bending over, or doing headstands immediately after meals, decreasing or discontinuing tobacco, alcohol, and carminative can be helpful. Elevation of the head of the bed, not with pillows but with wood blocks under the legs at the head of bed as long as it is not a waterbed can be useful.

Antacids and mucosal protectants such as alginic acid or sucralfate can also be helpful but have a more frequent dosing schedule. Prokinetic agents to enhance esophageal motility and tighten the lower esophageal sphincter can also be used. The oldest generic prokinetic Metoclopramide has a high incidence of central nervous system side effects and is now rarely used. Newer prokinetics have a safer profile.

A variety of endoscopic therapies have been developed, including procedures designed to reduce the lumen diameter to reduce reflux. Laparoscopic procedures using magnets and other implantable devices have also been utilized to create a physical barrier to the reflux of gastric contents into the esophagus. The standard surgical treatment for severe GERD is the Nissen fundoplication, where the upper part of the stomach is wrapped around the lower esophageal sphincter. This corrects the hiatal hernia by keeping the stomach and LES below the diaphragm preventing reflux. Medical therapy and surgical therapies appear to be equally effective for this often-chronic condition.

Gastrointestinal Motility

Motilin

Motilin is a hormone secreted by endocrine M cells in the small intestine, especially in the duodenum and jejunum. It was named motilin because of its ability to stimulate gastric activity. Erythromycin and related antibiotics act as motilin agonists, and are sometimes used for their ability to stimulate gastrointestinal motility. Another hormone ghrelin can also induce motilin like effects.

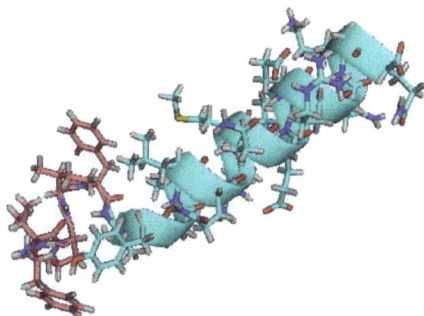

NMR solution structure of Motilin in phospholipid bicellar solution Author Adam Busch Pymol Structure Creative Commons License

Motilin triggers the migrating myoelectric complex component of gastrointestinal motility, which induces brief episodes of peristaltic activity several times an hour in between meals. Contractions of the gastric fundus and antrum triggered by motilin can cause stomach rumble or growls, borborygmi, and cramp like discomfort often described as hunger pains since they occur during a fasting period. The gastric emptying and peristaltic sweeping action clearing the stomach and small bowel of food residue or chyme has earned Motilin the moniker 'housekeeper of the gut'.

Gastrointestinal Pacemaker Cells

Interstitial cells of Cajal are pacemaker cells similar to the pacemaker cells of the heart, which cause the heart to beat regularly. They are present in the wall of the gut and communicate between the nervous system and the smooth muscle of the gut wall (Figure 1). When the signal arrives from the nervous system to the interstitial cells of Cajal that a person has eaten they begin their pacemaker function. This results in a coordinated and rhythmic set of contractions of the gut known as peristalsis, which propels food along the entire length of the digestive tract. The interstitial cells of Cajal were studied in relative obscurity for over one hundred years until the discovery that gastrointestinal stromal tumors (GIST) arise from interstitial cells of Cajal or an interstitial cell of Cajal-like precursor cell.

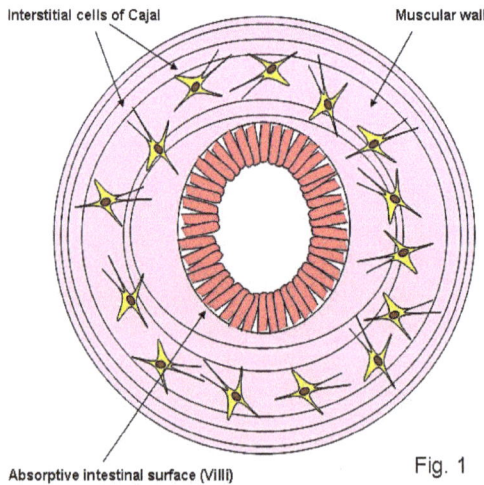

Fig. 1

liferaftgroup.org/wp Creative Commons License

Interstitial cell of Cajal are also thought to be the cells from which gastrointestinal stromal tumors (GISTs) arise. The interstitial cells of Cajal are derived from the mesoderm of the gastrointestinal tract and serves as a pacemaker for the peristaltic contractions of the smooth muscle. The interstitial cells of Cajal are named after Santiago Ramón y Cajal (1852 - 1934) a Spanish pathologist and Nobel laureate who was considered by many as the father of neuroscience.

The frequency of interstitial cell of Cajal pacemaker activity differs in different regions of the GI tract, 3 per minute in the stomach, twelve per minute in the duodenum, ten per minute in the ileum, and three per minute again in the colon. The loss of interstitial cells of Cajal may interrupt normal neural control of gastrointestinal contractions and lead to functional GI disorders, such as irritable bowel syndrome and chronic intestinal pseudo-obstruction. Diabetes mellitus often leads to gastrointestinal motility disorders.

Gastrointestinal motility disorders are a major source of morbidity and can have a profound influence on the quality of life. Irritable bowel syndrome is one of the most common of gastrointestinal disorders. Its prevalence in various countries around the world is between six and forty-six percent of the population. In the United States an estimated forty million people have the condition

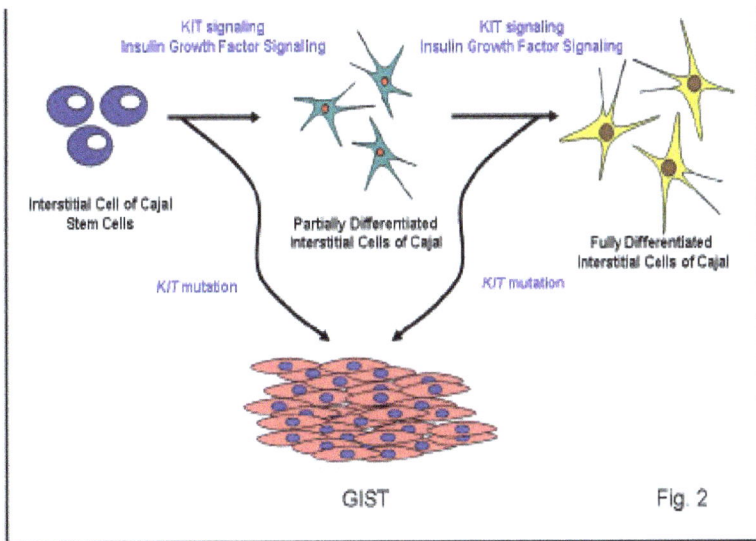

Pathway of interstitial cell of Cajal maturation and GIST formation. Interstitial cell of Cajal stem cells mature to partially differentiated and later fully differentiated interstitial cells of Cajal under the influence of KIT signaling and insulin growth factor signaling and likely many other growth and development factors. KIT or mutation in other genes such as platelet-derived growth factor receptor A leads to GIST formation.

ftgroup.org/wp Creative Commons License

Rapid Gastric Emptying

Rapid gastric emptying, also called dumping syndrome, occurs when undigested food empties too quickly into the small intestine. Early rapid gastric emptying begins during or right after a meal. Symptoms include nausea, vomiting, bloating, cramping, diarrhea, dizziness, and fatigue. Late rapid gastric emptying occurs 1 to 3 hours after eating. Symptoms include hypoglycemia (low blood sugar), weakness, sweating, and dizziness.

DUMPING SYNDROME

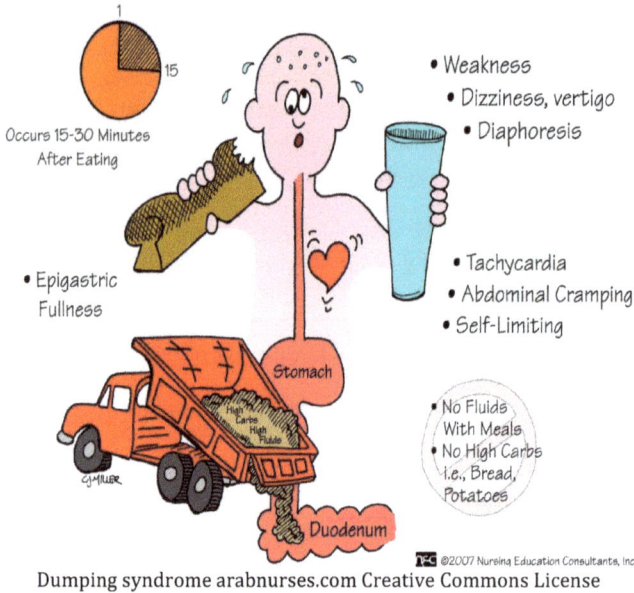

Occurs 15-30 Minutes After Eating

• Weakness
  • Dizziness, vertigo
  • Diaphoresis

• Tachycardia
• Abdominal Cramping
• Self-Limiting

• Epigastric Fullness

Stomach

• No Fluids With Meals
• No High Carbs i.e., Bread, Potatoes

Duodenum

©2007 Nursing Education Consultants, Inc.

Dumping syndrome arabnurses.com Creative Commons License

Rapid gastric emptying is usually the result of stomach surgery such as fundoplication or gastric bypass. The condition is also seen in people with Zollinger-Ellison syndrome, a rare disorder involving a gastrin hormone-secreting tumor in the pancreas. Treatment of rapid gastric emptying focuses on the underlying cause and may include changes in eating habits and medication. People who have the condition should eat several small meals a day that are low in carbohydrates. They should also drink liquids between meals and not with them. Prescription medications may also be utilized, with surgery as a last resort.

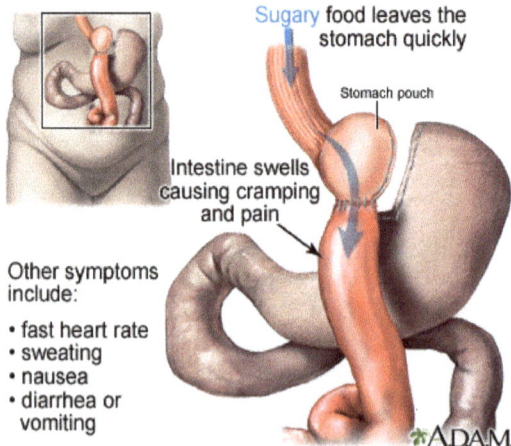

Sugary food leaves the stomach quickly

Stomach pouch

Intestine swells causing cramping and pain

Other symptoms include:

• fast heart rate
• sweating
• nausea
• diarrhea or vomiting

ADAM.

www.nlm.nih.gov Creative Commons License

Gastrointestinal Transit Time

Gastrointestinal transit time is the time period from ingestion of food or a biomarker until its elimination and exit from the digestive tract. The time period is highly variable and can be influenced by many factors including diet, physical activity, infection, inflammation, pharmaceuticals, etc. The gastrointestinal transit time can also be divided into the three subsets of gastric emptying, small intestinal transit and colonic transit.

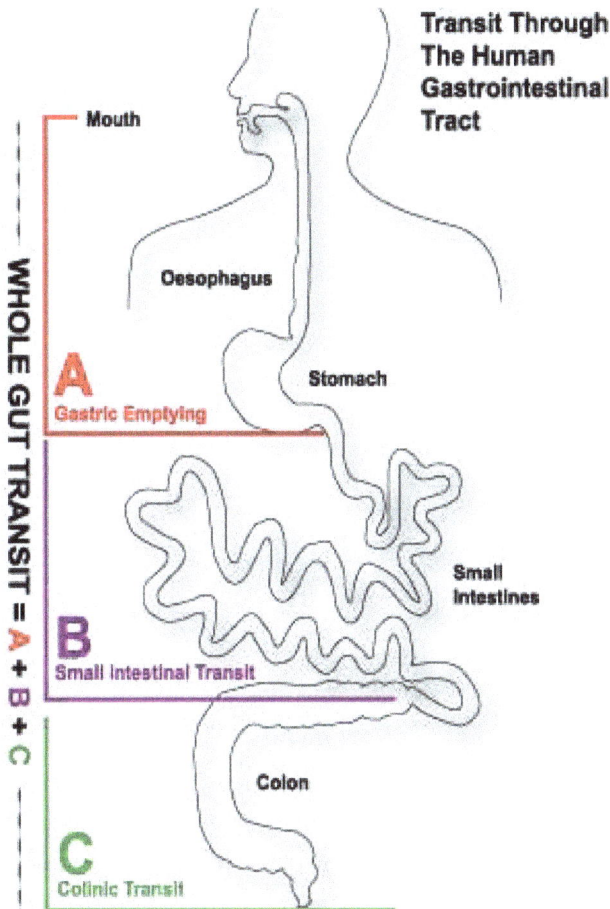

www.ibsresearchupdate.org Creative Commons License

The transit time is the general period of time it takes, from the swallow of ingestion to the elimination at defecation, for food to pass through the gastrointestinal track. Normal ranges are from half a day to two days but individuals vary. Certain conditions especially those with diarrhea may have a more rapid transit time, while those with neurologic conditions or diabetes may have a slow transit time.

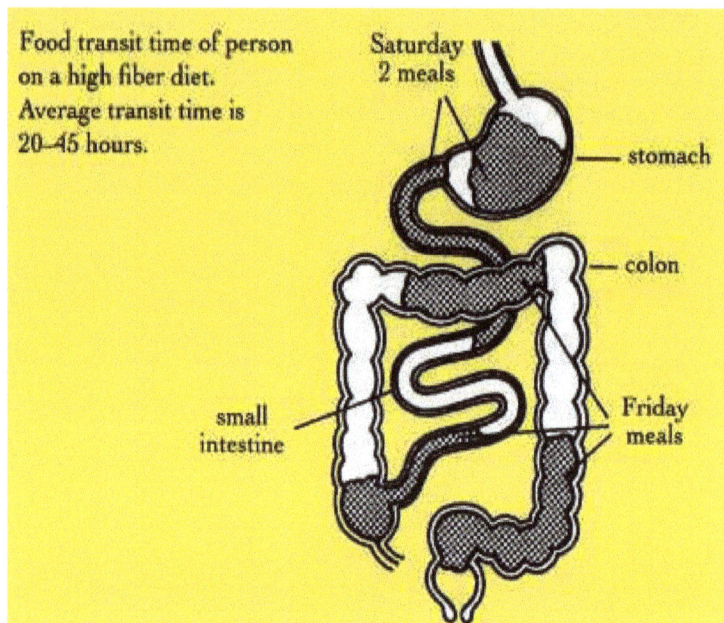

Food transit time of person on a high fiber diet. Average transit time is 20–45 hours.

Saturday 2 meals

stomach

colon

small intestine

Friday meals

www.elclorurodemagnesio.com Creative Commons License

In general it takes about one hour for half of the gastric contents to be processed and advanced into the duodenum and the stomach us usually empty two hours after ingestion. Approximately two to four hours is involved in digestion and absorption before the chyme is released into the colon for water absorption and packaging as feces. The material is eliminated approximately twelve to forty eight hours after ingestion.

Diabetics are particularly prone to a condition called gastroparesis, where the delay is primarily in gastric emptying. Although it is not uncommon to see certain undigested foods passed, like kernels of corn, more undigested foods may be seen with a rapid gut transit time.

Gastroparesis

Diabetes mellitus is one of the most common causes of delayed gastric emptying known as gastroparesis diabeticorum. It can also lead to generalized gastrointestinal motility disorder with delayed total gut transit times. Irritable bowel syndrome is also associated with gastrointestinal motility disorder.

This disorder of delayed gastric emptying is most often seen as a consequence of neuropathy secondary to diabetes mellitus. The delayed gastric emptying prevents both the nutritional intake as well as swallowed gasses from leaving the stomach. Meals that are high in fat cause the release of hormones that slows down gut motility and delays gastric emptying.

This can lead to increased burping and belching as well as distension. Side effects from medications, especially narcotic analgesics, and antidepressants are well-recognized causes of delayed gastrointestinal peristalsis and bloating. There are a number of pharmacological agents that have prokinetic actions that may be of value in treating delayed gastric emptying.

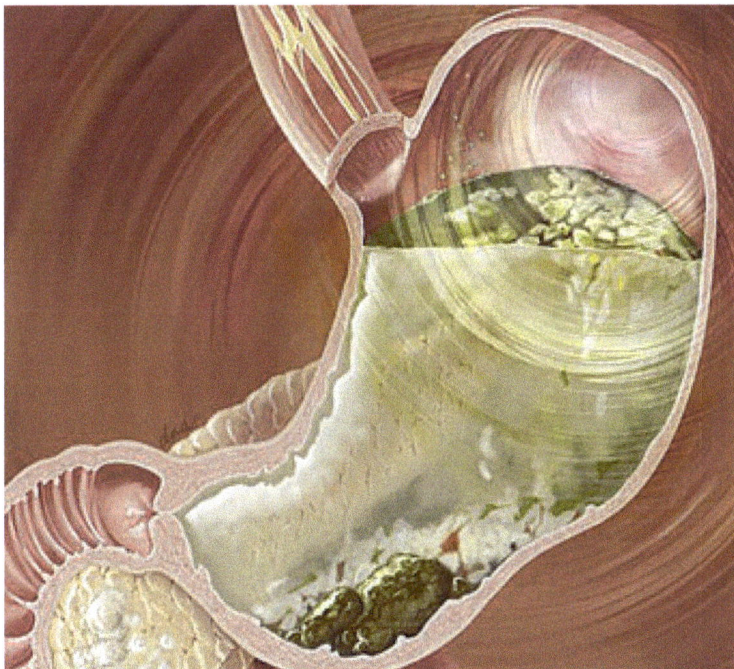

Gastroparesis is the delayed physiological emptying of the stomach with solids and liquids accumulating leading to discomfort, bloating, and distension and belching. Creative Commons License

Peristalsis & Segmental Contractions

Peristalsis (Greek peri-, "around" and stallein, "to place") is the propulsive wave of muscular contraction and relaxation, which advances digestive material through the intestinal tract. Earthworms use a similar mechanism in their movement. The process of peristalsis is controlled by the medulla oblongata of the brainstem. Segmental contractions are used to mix the chime with digestive juices and enzymes and to bring additional nutrient material in contact with the villi and microvilli of the small bowel mucosa.

Digestive material in the stomach is called chyme that in the esophagus and small intestine is called a bolus. The peristaltic wave in the esophagus advances the bolus in a wave lasting less than ten seconds. In the small intestine peristaltic waves lasts for a few seconds and the bolus is advanced a few centimeters. It serves to mix the chyme as digestion and absorption of nutrients occurs during the transit through the small intestine.

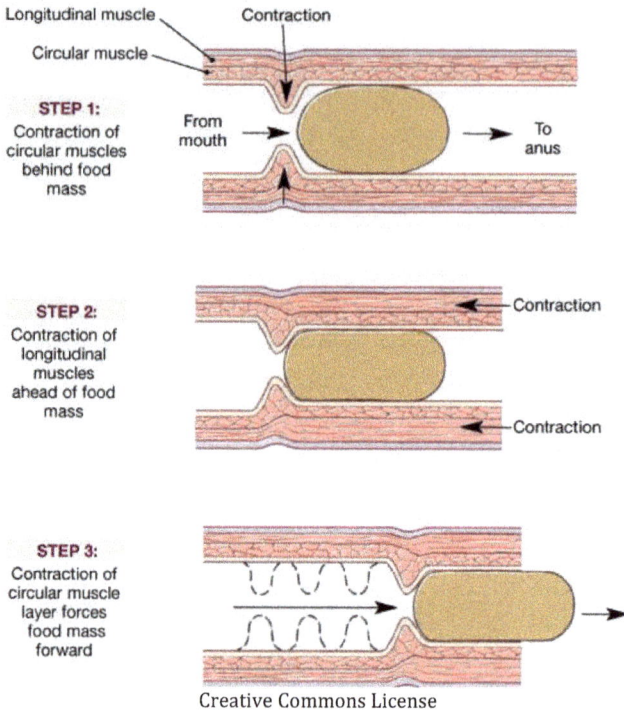

Longitudinal muscle   Contraction

Circular muscle

STEP 1:
Contraction of
circular muscles
behind food
mass

From
mouth   To
anus

STEP 2:
Contraction of
longitudinal
muscles
ahead of food
mass

Contraction

Contraction

STEP 3:
Contraction of
circular muscle
layer forces
food mass
forward

Creative Commons License

Migrating motor complexes (MMC) are waves of gastric emptying followed by peristaltic activity that sweep through the stomach and small intestines in between meals. They each last for a moment or two and occur in a cyclic pattern several times an hour, advancing any remaining food residue or chyme through the small intestine into the colon. The maintenance of regular peristaltic activity during meals and intermittently during fasting is also thought to prevent the migration of colonic bacteria into the terminal Ileum.

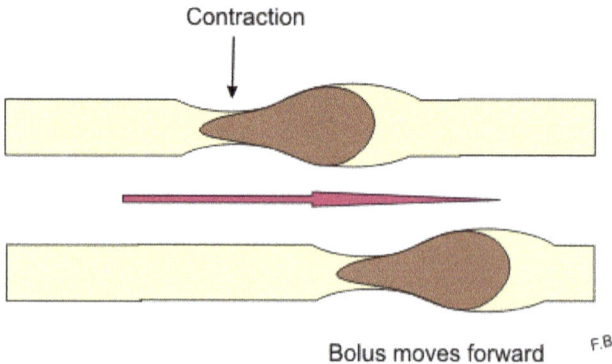

Contraction

Bolus moves forward   F.B

Peristaltic contractions in the gut. Author Boumphreyfr Creative Commons License

The hormone motilin triggers the MMC, as can motilin like agonists such as the antibiotic erythromycin. The at times audible borborygmi from the MMC are also referred to as stomach rumbles or growls and are also commonly thought of as hunger pains since the cramps occur during a fasting state.

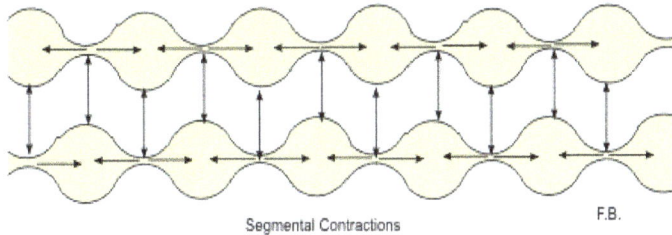

Segmental Contractions   F.B.

Segmental contractions in the gut. Author Boumphreyfr Creative Commons License

Gastrointestinal motility is also under the control of local enteric neurons that coordinate intestinal motility. Cholinergic neurons cause contraction and shortening of the circular muscle layer, shortening of longitudinal muscle, distension of the intestine. As chyme enters the duodenum, carbohydrates and proteins are only partially digested, no fat digestion has taken place. Digestion continues in the small intestine where hypertonic chyme has a low acidic pH and mixing is required for the enzymes and substrates to interact.

The most common motion of the small intestine is the motility action called segmentation. It is initiated by intrinsic pacemaker cells (Cajal cells) with the segmentation mixing the contents while peristaltic activity moves the bolus distally towards the ileocecal valve. After the bulk of the nutrients have been absorbed the gastroileal reflex and gastrin relax the ileocecal sphincter and allow chyme to pass into the large intestine. The colon absorbs the water and electrolytes from the still liquid chyme that is increasingly solidified by water absorption as it transits the large intestine.

Mass Movement

The large intestine (colon) does not have peristaltic activity like the small intestine illustrated above. Feces are propelled through the large intestine by mass movements, which occur one to three times per day. The stool stored in the rectum is expelled via the anus by defecation. Haustral contractions are slow segmenting movements that move the contents of the colon by peristaltic activity towards the rectum.. The haustra sequentially contract as they are stimulated by distension.

The defecation reflex is triggered by distension of rectal walls by feces. When stimulated the defecation reflex contracts the rectal walls and relaxes the internal anal sphincter. Voluntary signals stimulate relaxation of the external anal sphincter and defecation occurs.

Gastrointestinal Tract

The gastrointestinal tract is also known as the alimentary tract or alimentary canal. It consists of the esophagus, stomach, small intestine and large intestine. It may be considered to be the continuous passageway of the hollow viscous organs, from the mouth to the anus. It is also known as the digestive, intestinal, gastrointestinal, or GI tract. The gastrointestinal system is an expanded entity that includes structures other than the hollow viscus.

The gastrointestinal system includes the accessory organs necessary for digestion, such as the salivary glands, pancreas, liver, gallbladder, and their associated ducts. In an adult male human, the alimentary tract is twenty feet (five meters) long in a living subject. If the alimentary tract is measured at autopsy its length may be increased up to thirty feet (nine meters) because of the loss of the muscular tone and peristaltic contractions

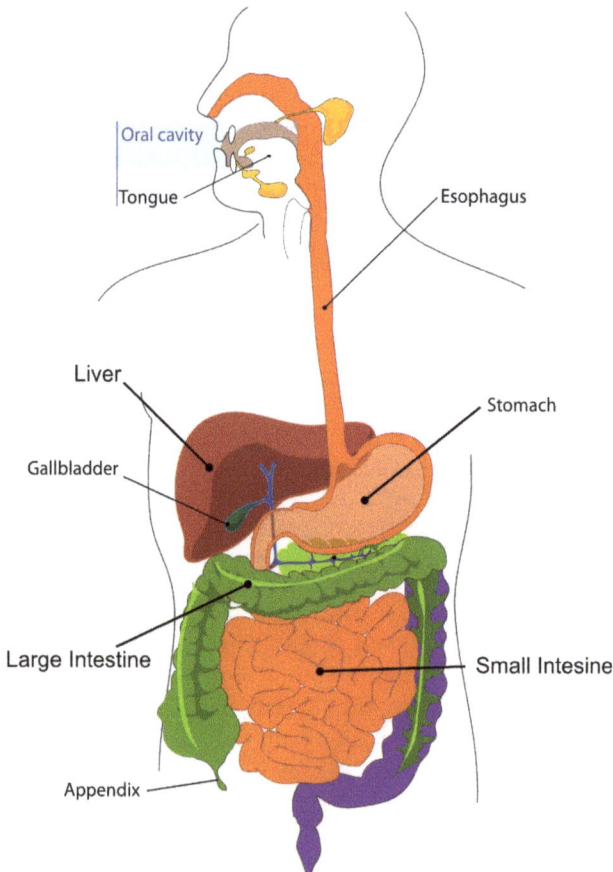

Digestive System. Creative Commons License

The alimentary tract may also be delineated as three distinct regions,

the foregut, midgut, and hindgut. This terminology reflects the embryological origin of each segment of the tract. The tissue of the gut actively secretes and releases hormones that help to regulate the digestive process. The long recognized gastrointestinal hormones, including gastrin, secretin, cholecystokinin, have now been joined by more recently discovered hormones. These include leptin, ghrelin, bombesin, neuropeptide Y and others that are mediated through either intracrine or autocrine mechanisms. The multiple hormones may have individual effects, as well as acting with their counterparts in both positive and negative feedback loops. They have powerful effects not only on the digestive tract, but also on the brain and enteric nervous system. They have a profound influence on the satiety center, the area of the brain that plays a vital function in the control of appetite and weight.

The upper alimentary tract consists of the esophagus, stomach, and duodenum. The ligament of Treitz is considered the anatomical landmark that serves as the dividing line between the upper and lower alimentary tracts. The lower alimentary tract includes most of the small intestine, including the jejunum and ileum. The lower alimentary tract also includes all of the large intestine, consisting of the appendix, cecum, ascending colon, transverse colon, descending colon, sigmoid colon, rectum, and anus. The intestines may also commonly be referred to as the alimentary tract, alimentary canal, digestive tract, gastrointestinal (GI) tract, bowels, small bowel, large bowel, hollow viscus, gut, entrails, viscera, or innards. The lumen is the hollow distensible cavity where digestion and absorption take place.

The swallowed food is described as a bolus as it leaves the mouth. When the bolus leaves the stomach and exits through the pyloric sphincter and enters into the duodenum it is now known as chime. The chime has already been partially digested by salivary and gastric enzymes and acids, as well as having gone through a churning and mixing process in the stomach. When the chime leaves the last portion of the small intestine, known as the ileum, it passes through the ileocecal valve. Once it has passed through the ileocecal valve it has entered the cecum, the first portion of the colon, also known as the large intestine or large bowel. The material, which was known as chime on the small intestine side of the ileocecal valve, is now described as feces as it has entered into the colon. The major function of the colon is the absorption of water from the liquid feces that enters the cecum.

As the water is absorbed through the colonic epithelium the feces is solidified and finally stored in the rectum until defecation and elimination take place. The absorption of water is important to conserve the body's fluid balance and maintain adequate hydration. If too little water is absorbed from the feces it may remain liquid or loose and contribute to diarrhea. If excess water removal takes place the feces can become firm and difficult to eliminate resulting in constipation.

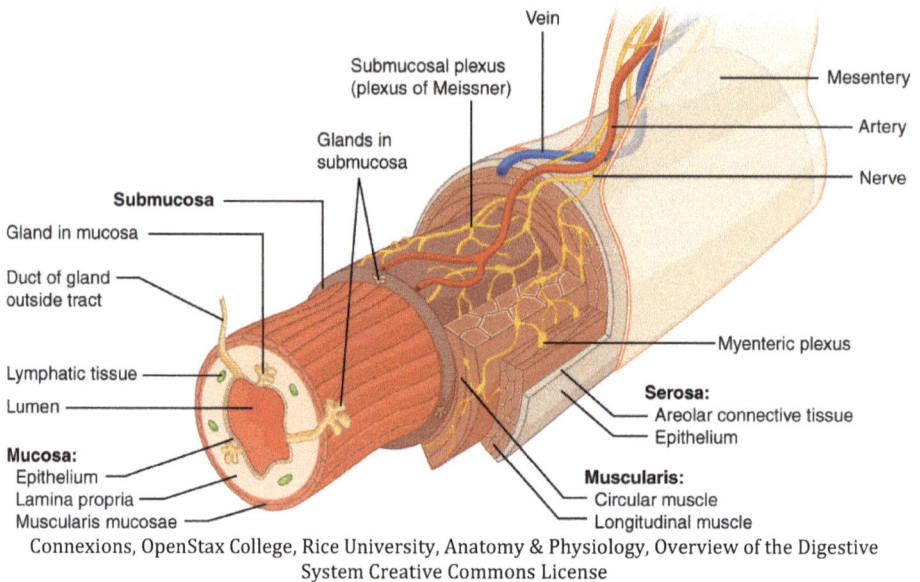

Connexions, OpenStax College, Rice University, Anatomy & Physiology, Overview of the Digestive System Creative Commons License

Going from the inside of the lumen towards the outer wall, there are several layers of tissue found in the anatomy of the gastrointestinal organs. The layers of the intestine, starting from the lumen, includes the mucosa (glandular epithelium and muscularis mucosa), sub mucosa, muscularis externa (made up of inner circular and outer longitudinal muscles), and the covering serosa. The sensory nerve fibers of the small intestine and colon can sense distension and spasm, but not other pain sensations such as those that would normally be felt by the skin if cut or burned.

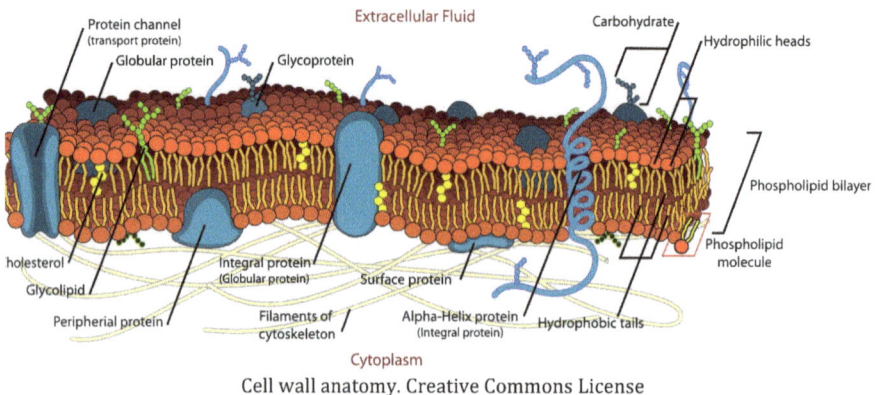

Cell wall anatomy. Creative Commons License

The small intestine is divided into three anatomical segments. The short first portion is immediately distal to the pyloric sphincter, the valve that empties the stomach. This first portion of the duodenum following the stomach is called the duodenum. The term duodenum comes from the middle Latin phrase, duodenum digitorium "space of twelve digits,". A translation of the Greek dodekadaktylon, literally "twelve fingers long," was described by the Greek physician Herophilus (c. 353-280).

The first portion of the duodenum has the critical function of receiving the highly acidic gastric contents. It secretes sodium bicarbonate to neutralize the potent stomach acid. Without its natural ability to neutralize gastric acid, the duodenal mucosa may become injured or inflamed, possibly resulting in an ulcer and internal bleeding.

Brunner glands (Duodenal glands) are secretory compound tubular submucosal glands. They are commonly found in the proximal duodenum. The main function of Brunner glands is to produce mucus and an alkaline solution containing sodium bicarbonate. It protects the duodenal mucosa from the potent gastric acid and neutralizes the chyme leaving the stomach and entering the duodenum Brunner's glands also secrete the polypeptide hormone urogastrone. Urogastrone inhibits the gastric parietal and chief cells from secreting hydrochloric acid and as well as their digestive enzymes. The hormone was given the name urogastrone because it can be identified and isolated from the urine as a fluorescent pigment. The hormonal structure is derived from epidermal growth factor.

Additional quantities of sodium bicarbonate enter into the second portion of the duodenum after being secreted by the pancreas. The pancreatic duct, as well as the bile duct, typically enter the second portion of the duodenum together. They enter the duodenum via an anatomical structure called the Ampulla of Vater. Within the Ampulla of Vater is a muscular valve known as the Sphincter of Oddi. The Sphincter of Oddi controls the flow of bile and pancreatic juice into the duodenum. The bile is produced in the liver and may be stored in the gallbladder for later release as needed. The pancreas also produces and secretes digestive enzymes, in addition to the sodium bicarbonate it secretes to neutralize gastric acid.

The neutralized chime is mixed with the potent digestive enzymes and bile furthering the digestive process and preparing nutrients for absorption.. The jejunum, the middle portion of the small intestine between the duodenum and the ileum, was given its name after the Latin word jējūnus, which means empty or poor, so called because it was always thought to be empty after death.

The ileum, from the Latin Ilium meaning flank or groin, is the final segment of the small intestine and enters the cecum of the colon close to the appendix at the ileocecal valve. The small intestine is described as small because the lumen is narrower than the lumen of the large intestine. The average length of the small intestine is twenty-three feet (seven meters) and is approximately one inch (two and one half centimeters) in diameter. It is substantially longer than the approximately five-foot length of the large intestine, also called the colon.

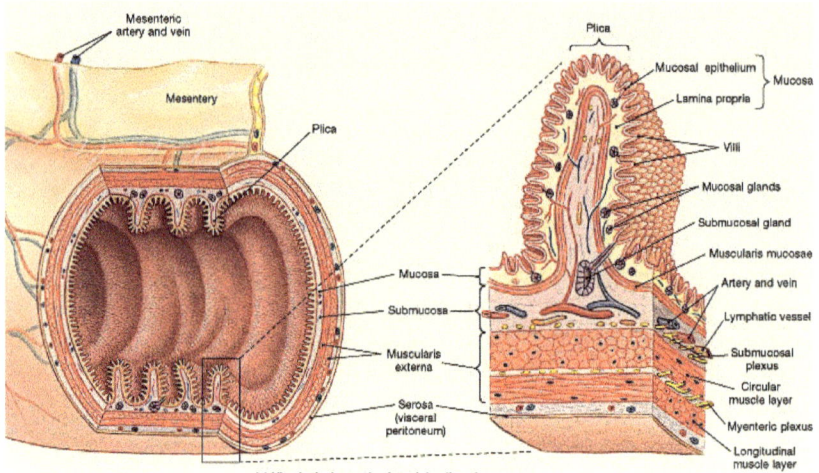

(a) Histological organization of the digestive tract
Creative Commons License

In spite of the relatively long length of the small intestine, its absorptive capacity would not be sufficient to maintain nutrition for an organism the size of humans, if it were a simple hollow tube. Without modifications to increase its surface area, the nutritional needs of a large mammal such as humans would exceed its absorptive ability. The small intestine has several remarkable features that dramatically increase its absorptive capacity. These consist of deep circular folds of the mucosa and sub mucosa known as plica circulares or plica. These folds work in conjunction with millions of fingerlike extensions of the mucosa called villi.

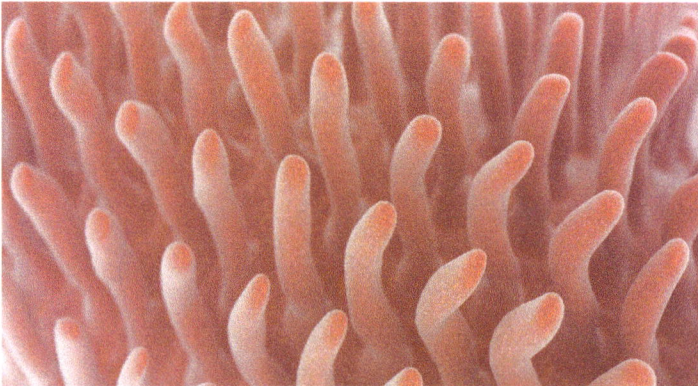

Villi increase the surface area for absorption. Creative Commons License

These villi are provided with additional microscopic projections of the mucosal cell plasma membranes called microvilli. Each of these modifications dramatically increases the surface area available to meet the nutritional needs of larger animals such as humans.. The surface area available to the average human adult for digestive processes, enzymatic activity, and absorption exceeds that of a championship tennis court.

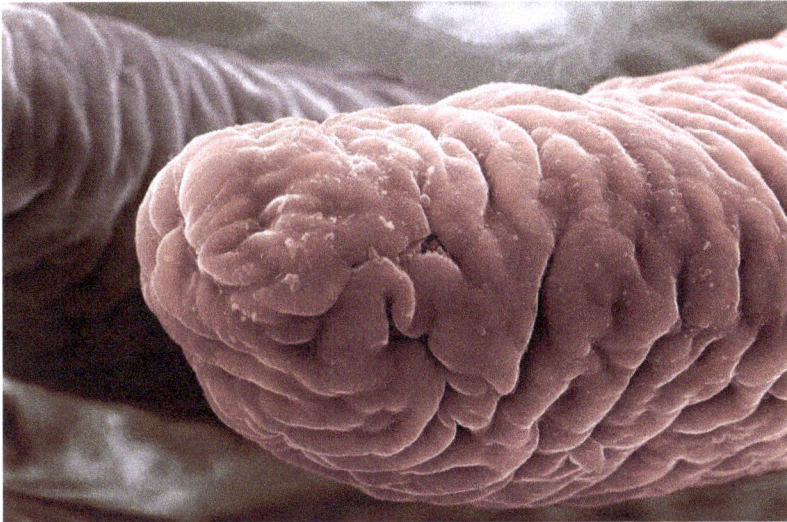

wellcomeimages.org Close up of intestinal villi Creative Commons License

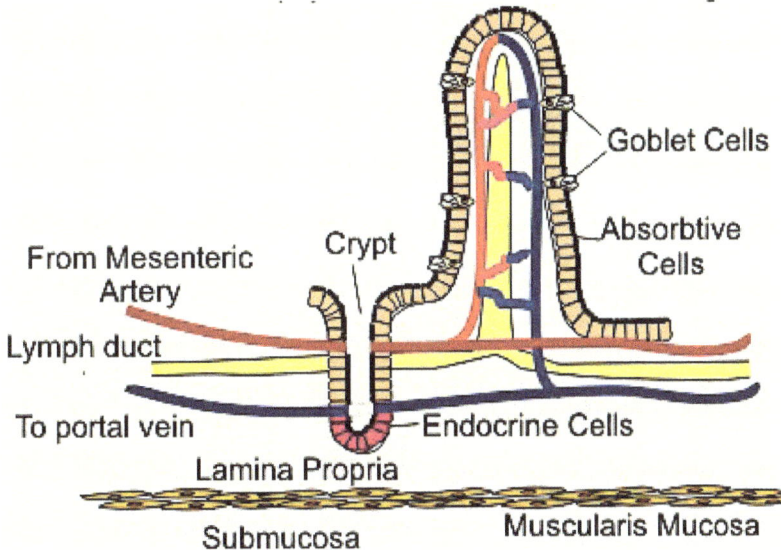

Goblet Cells

Absorbtive Cells

From Mesenteric Artery

Crypt

Lymph duct

To portal vein

Endocrine Cells

Lamina Propria

Submucosa

Muscularis Mucosa

Diagrammatic anatomy of a villous. Wikibooks Gastrointestinal Physiology Frank Boumphrey, MD Creative Commons License

The small intestinal mucosal epithelial cells consist of absorptive cells, mucus secreting goblet cells, entero-endocrine cells that secrete gastrointestinal hormones, and interspersed intraepithelial lymphocytes and T cells. The lymphocytes and T cells are important in the immune response, as the gut is exposed to the vast majority of foreign pathogens introduced into the body.

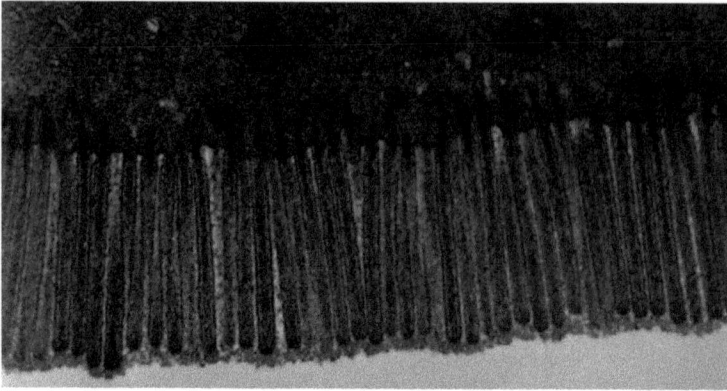

Each villous has thousands of microvilli, as demonstrated on this scanning Transmission electron microscope image of a human jejunal epithelial cell. Image shows absorptive cell with the densely packed microvilli that make up the absorptive border. Eac Louisa Howard, Katherine Connolly Creative Commons License

There is growing evidence that exposure to microorganisms during a normal childbirth leads to a healthy gut flora. Those who were delivered via a Caesarian section are more prone to a number of gastrointestinal disturbances as well as other systemic conditions. The microbiome are the microorganisms that live within our digestive tracts, on our skin, and in several regions on and in our body. The vast majority of these organisms are beneficial. They may provide active benefits, including supplying nutritional metabolic products that humans cannot manufacture. In addition these beneficial organisms, known as commensals, prevent pathogens from establishing colonies, which could lead to illness.

The cells of the intestinal crypts also secrete an intestinal juice in response to irritation of the mucosal lining. This solution is slightly alkaline and isotonic with blood plasma. It is predominantly water, with some mucus, and with very little enzymatic activity. A number of intestinal infections, toxins, or inflammatory processes may stimulate the release of intestinal juice, which may lead to diarrhea. The liquid chyme has over ninety percent of its nutritional value digested and absorbed by the small intestine. The chyme exits the small intestine via the ileocecal valve, entering into the cecum of the large intestine, also called the colon. The lumen of the gastrointestinal tract, although commonly thought of as being deep within the body, is actually contiguous with and exposed to the external environment. It is a potential pathway for pathogenic microorganisms. Peyer patches are lymphoid nodules located in the laminae propria layer of the mucosa and submucosa of the ileum. They are located only in the ileum and are not present in the duodenum or jejunum of the small intestine

There are approximately thirty Peyer patches, each a few centimeters long. They are involved in the immune surveillance of the gastrointestinal tract and have a response and defense mechanism Peyer patches are covered by specialized epithelial cells called microfold cells (M cells). They contain B and T lymphocytes and are an important feature of the gastrointestinal immune response. The cells of Peyer patches allow the sampling of antigens in the gut lumen. The antigen may stimulate a response from the Peyer patches T cells, B cell lymphocytes, and memory cells. Activated lymphocytes may stimulate and magnify the immune response. They can pass into the mesenteric lymph nodes and travel via the lymphatic thoracic duct into the blood stream. From there, they may circulate throughout the gastrointestinal tract as a defense.

Pathogenic microorganisms and other antigens that enter the intestinal tract may encounter several layers of the body's immune defense. Besides the B-lymphocytes, and T-lymphocytes from Peyer patches, the antigen may also encounter macrophages, and dendritic cells. The Mucosa Associated Lymphoid Tissue (MALT) also provides immunological defenses. If injured, the ability of the small bowel to digest and absorb nutrients may be compromised. A condition that temporarily damages the small intestine, like diarrhea from a viral or bacterial gastroenteritis, often called a stomach flu, can cause a blunting or shortening of the villi. This decreases the absorptive capacity of the small intestine and may lead to diarrhea.

The damage to the villi will also lead to the loss of digestive enzymes that reside on the villi. This is one of the reasons people are often advised to avoid dairy products for a week or so after stomach flu. The villi need time to recover and return enzyme levels to normal. If you eat or drink lactose without waiting until the recovery is complete, you may end up with symptoms of lactose intolerance such as gas and diarrhea.

When the liquid chyme leaves the jejunum and ileum of the small intestine, it goes through the ileocecal valve and becomes feces. In the cecum of the colon lies the infamous appendix, which for thousands of years was a mystery as to its purpose. Its function has only very recently been identified. It stores as a reservoir of intestinal bacteria, representing the healthy gut microbiome, from which the gut flora can be replenished after a bout of intestinal dysentery. The gut microbiome is much more important than most people, including physicians and research scientists, have given it credit for. The microbes of the body far outnumber the number of human cells. The vast majority are commensals, and are engaged with us in a symbiotic relationship from which we both benefit.

The colon, unlike the small intestine, is less involved in the digestion of foods and nutrients. It is primarily involved in the absorption of water and sodium, as well as the absorption of some fat-soluble vitamins such as vitamin K. The colon removes the excess moisture from the watery chyme, and the stool solidifies as it transits the gut. It is stored in the rectum and sigmoid colon, awaiting the right opportunity to be eliminated through defecation. A process or illness that impairs the colon's absorption of water will lead to more fluid stool and diarrhea. If the elimination is delayed moisture continues to be absorbed and the stools can become harder resulting in constipation. The colon is not a vital organ, and people can live a normal life span without it, in spite of the challenges of avoiding dehydration.

Global Warming

Global warming due to greenhouse gas production from human activity is mainly due to deforestation, the combustion of fossil fuels, livestock enteric fermentation and manure management, and landfill emissions. In terms of biomass bacteria would be the main contributors to global warming by their methane production. Other contenders nominated have been termites, which have over 2000 species and are prolific methane producers (initial reports suggested that they produce 40% of global methane), livestock such as cows, sheep, and pigs, and lastly dinosaurs, which are no longer around to defend their reputations.

A ruminant (Latin *ruminare* - to chew over again) is a mammal that digests plants in a multi compartment stomach through bacterial fermentation. It regurgitates the semi-digested mass, called cud, and chews it again and repeats the swallow. The process of re-chewing the cud is called "ruminating". There are about 150 species of ruminants, which include both domestic and wild species. Ruminating mammals include cattle, goats, sheep, giraffes, yaks, deer, camels, llamas, and antelope. Ruminant bacterial fermentation is a significant contributor to global methane production, which is over twenty times as potent a greenhouse gas as carbon dioxide. To incentivize efforts to reduce livestock methane production a number of countries have proposed taxes on the release of greenhouse gasses.

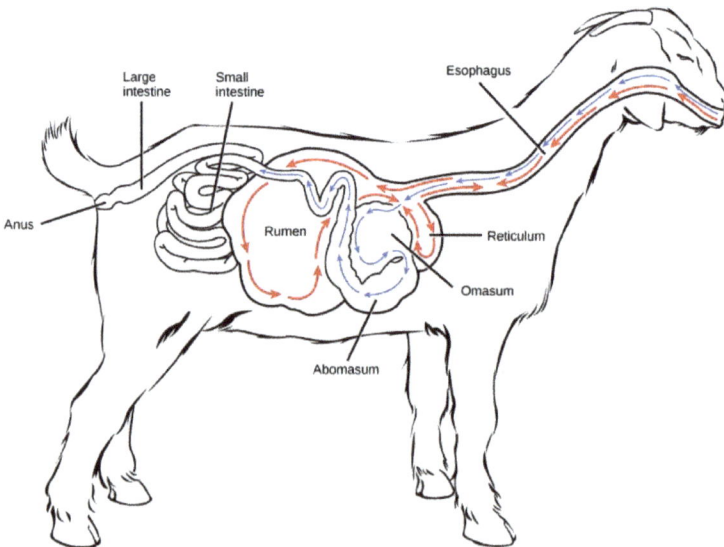

www.rice.edu Creative Commons License

It took extensive scientific experimentation to collect the intestinal gasses of herds of cattle before it was discovered that the methane production was coming from the other end of the cows and other ruminants. It is the burps and belches from the multi compartment ruminant stomach that is the primary source of methane. The Great Chicago Fire, which destroyed the city in 1871, has traditionally been blamed on Mrs. O'Leary's cow kicking over a kerosene lamp. With the large volume of methane produced it is just as likely to have been caused by her cow farting and belching,. But that would not have been an acceptable cause in Victorian times.

Kangaroos are herbivores and as marsupial their burps and farts contain little or no methane, a potent greenhouse gas. It appears that the reduced methane emissions are due to the microbes in the kangaroos' gut flora. Australian researchers hope that introducing a similar gut flora to other methane producing herbivores such as cattle and sheep will contribute to a reduction in greenhouse gasses and the resultant global warming. Methane can cause about 20 times as much atmospheric warming as an equivalent volume of carbon dioxide.

Kangaroos, like cattle and sheep, are ruminants that re-chew their cud with the assistance of the gut flora to digest the and metabolize their cellulose based grazing diet. In the foregut the meal is broken down by fermentation with carbon dioxide and hydrogen released. In cows and other ruminants, microbes called methanogens transform these gases into methane. But in the kangaroos' guts the same hydrogen and carbon dioxide may be utilized by bacteria called acetogens to produce acetate, a volatile fatty acid.

These microbes compete with methanogens to use the carbon dioxide and hydrogen, so the more acetogens the less methane production. The odds are in generally in favor of methanogens, since the process of methane production is generally more energy efficient than producing acetate. One of the acetogen microbes, *Blautia coccoides,* live in cows as well as in kangaroos. Further research is being undertaken to understand why the organism is more successful in competing with the methanogens in kangaroos than in other herbivores.

Carbon dioxide, methane, nitrous oxide, and three groups of fluorinated gases (sulfur hexafluoride, hydro fluorocarbons , and per fluorocarbons) are the major greenhouse gases impacted by human activity. These are regulated under the Kyoto Protocol an international treaty that was adopted in 2005. Nitrogen dioxide (NO_2) warms the atmosphere three hundred and ten times more than carbon dioxide, and methane twenty-one times more than carbon dioxide. Although CFCs are greenhouse gases, regulations were initiated because CFCs' cause ozone depletion, not because of their contribution to global warming. Ozone depletion itself has a relatively minor effect on greenhouse warming.

Dinosaurs are no longer around to defend themselves and have been accused of contributing to global warming. We do not know if they were ruminants and contributed by belching up gasses as well, but there should be no doubt that they were big time farters. Their nickname "thunder lizards" may have more to do with their farts than their footsteps.

Gluten

Gluten (Latin gluten, "glue") is a protein composite of gliadin and glutenin found conjoined with starch in the endosperm of various grass grains related to wheat, and some forms of oats. In barley the gluten component is known as hordein, in rye it is known as secalin. Corn, maize, and rice do not contain gluten. Gluten gives elasticity to dough and gives the final product a chewy texture. Bread flours are high in gluten (hard wheat); pastry flours have a lower gluten content. Kneading promotes the chewiness of a product by the formation of gluten strands and cross-links. In wheat, alpha-gliadins are not only seed storage proteins, but also act as inhibitors of alpha-amylase activity. About 1 in 133 people in developed nations have sensitivity reactions to gluten, which can damage the villi and microvilli of the small intestine. This can lead to malabsorption, gas, diarrhea, and a variety of metabolic disorders and physical ailments. The treatment is a strict gluten free diet.

Buddhist monks discovered gluten in the 7th century. The monks, who were vegetarians, were trying to find a substitute for meat. They discovered that when they submerged dough in water, the starch washed off and all that was left was a meat-like, textured, gummy mass, the gluten. Gluten sensitivity as the cause of Celiac Disease was discovered during the World War Two occupation of the Netherlands where celiac patients actually improved when all of the wheat was confiscated by Nazi Germany for their military.

Gluten, a substance in wheat and other grains,
may be found in a variety of foods including
breads, cakes, cereals, pasta, commercial dairy
products and alcoholic beverages

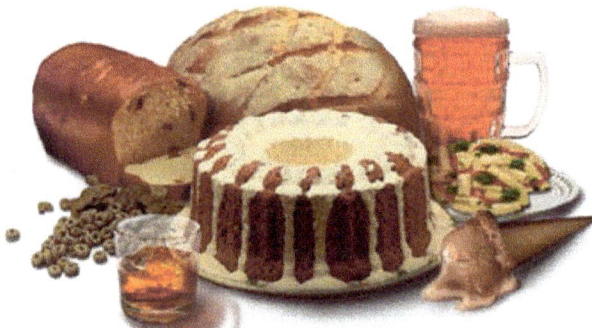

digestivedisease.uthscsa.edu Creative Commons License

Gluten Sensitive Enteropathy

Gluten Sensitive Enteropathy is also known by a number of other names, including, Celiac Sprue, Celiac Disease, Sprue, and Non-Tropical Sprue. It is not synonymous with gluten intolerance although it may be considered a more severe form of intolerance leading to physical and physiological changes in the gut and other areas of the body.

Celiac (Greek κοιλιακός (koiliakós, "abdominal") disease is an autoimmune disorder of the small intestine that occurs in genetically predisposed people and is thought to occur in up to 1% of United States population. It may also be called celiac sprue, nontropical sprue, endemic sprue, sprue, gluten enteropathy, gluten-sensitive enteropathy, and gluten intolerance. It is caused by a reaction to gliadin, a prolamin protein of gluten, found in wheat, rye, barley, and sometimes oats.

Humans first started to cultivate grains in the Fertile Crescent of Western Asia about 9500 BCE) it is probable that coeliac disease did not occur before this time. Aretaeus of Cappadocia, living in the second century described a malabsorptive syndrome presumed to be celiac disease with pain, flatulence, and a malodorous intractable diarrhea. While a role for carbohydrates had been suspected, the link with wheat was not made until the 1940's by the Dutch pediatrician Dr. Willem Karel Dicke. He noticed that during the Dutch famine of 1944 the scarcity of wheat and bread led the rate among children affected by CD to drop essentially zero, but returned to over 35% once wheat was again available after the war.

On exposure to gliadin the enzyme tissue transglutaminase modifies the protein triggering an immune response causes an inflammatory reaction in the small bowel. This leads to damage and atrophy of the villous lining of the small intestine that is critical for digestion and absorption of nutrients. Treatment requires a gluten free diet to avoid the offending protein. is a lifelong gluten-free diet.

Typical and Atypical Symptoms of Celiac Disease

Typical Symptoms

Abdominal distention	Failure to thrive
Chronic diarrhea	

Atypical Symptoms

Independent of malabsorption

Alopecia	Myasthenia gravis
Ataxia	Polyneuropathy
Dental enamel hypoplasia	Primary biliary cirrhosis
Dermatitis herpetiformis	Psoriasis
Dilative cardiomyopathy	Recurrent aphthous
Epilepsy	stomatitis
Hyperthyroidism	Recurrent pericarditis
Hypothyroidism	Vasculitis
Isolated hypertransaminasemia	

Secondary to malabsorption

Flatulence	Recurrent spontaneous
Hepatic stenosis	abortion
Osteopenia	Short stature
Recurrent abdominal pain	Sideropenic anemia

www.uspharmacist.com Creative Commons License

Celiac disease can present with malabsorption, steatorrhea weight loss, anemia, fatigue, and other symptoms related to the nutritional deficiencies. Milder or subclinical cases may present without symptoms, often discovered by abnormal results on a routine blood test. When chronic diarrhea is present in celiac disease it is often pale, voluminous, malodorous because of fat absorption leading to steatorrhea. Abdominal pain, cramping, bloating, distension, and gaseousness with mouth ulcers may be present. It is my unusual for lead patients to be seen and treated for irritable bowel or other conditions for several years before the correct diagnosis becomes apparent.

Untreated celiac disease has an increased risk of adenocarcinoma and lymphoma of the small bowel. Malabsorption may lead to nutritional deficiencies such as minerals and the fat-soluble vitamins A, D, E, and K. Anemia may develop from iron insufficiency as well as from deficiencies of folic acid and vitamin B_{12} which may give rise to megaloblastic anemia and neuropathy. Calcium and vitamin D malabsorption (and secondary hyperparathyroidism) may cause osteopenia (decreased mineral content of the bone) or osteoporosis. Vitamin K deficiency interferes with to the bloods ability to clot and can present as abnormal bleeding. Bacterial overgrowth of the small intestine can occur aggravating malabsorption or preventing the resolution of malabsorption with a gluten free diet.

A variety of other conditions, especially autoimmune disorders are more common in those with celiac disease. These include those IgA deficiency, dermatitis herpetiformis, diabetes mellitus, autoimmune thyroiditis, primary biliary cirrhosis, hyposplenism, and microscopic colitis, abnormal liver function tests, delayed growth and development., Addison disease (adrenal insufficiency), alopecia areata, Down syndrome (trisomy 21), osteoporosis, Sjögren syndrome, systemic lupus erythematosis, and Turner syndrome.

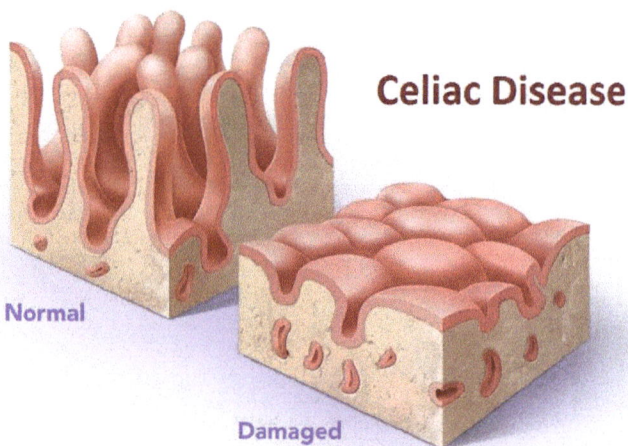

Intestinal villi in celiac disease are atrophic ih.constantcontact.com Creative Commons License

There are several tests that can be used to assist in diagnosis. The level of symptoms may determine the order of the tests, but all tests lose their usefulness if the person is already eating a gluten-free diet. Intestinal damage begins to heal within weeks of gluten being removed from the diet, and antibody levels decline over months. For those who have already started on a gluten-free diet, it may be necessary to perform a challenge with some gluten-containing food in one meal a day over 6 weeks before repeating the investigations.

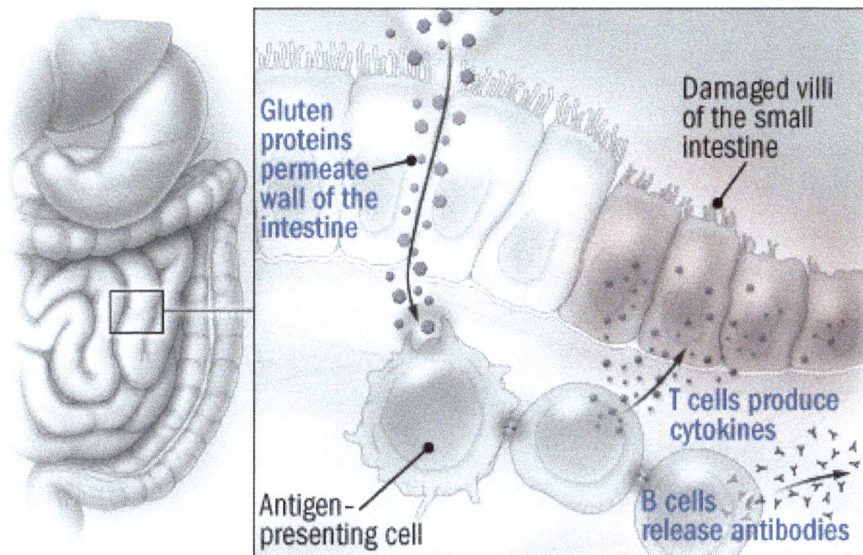

Gluten proteins permeate wall of the intestine

Damaged villi of the small intestine

T cells produce cytokines

Antigen-presenting cell

B cells release antibodies

www.health.harvard.edu Creative Commons License

Diagnostic tests are very accurate unless a gluten free diet was instituted before testing. The tests accuracy is diminished with longer time periods from gluten exposure. Serological blood tests have high sensitivity and specificity for celiac disease but endoscopy and small bowel biopsy is usually necessary for a definitive diagnosis of celiac disease. Anti-endomysial immunoglobulin A (IgA) antibodies and IgA tissue anti-transglutaminase (tTG) have over 90% sensitivity and nearly 99% specificity.

Gut-Brain-Microbiome-Food Axis

A relatively recent discovery has been that the gut brain axis has a very important third component, the microbiome. The gut microbiome is also known as the gut flora and consists of the multitude of other life forms residing within the gut. These include bacteria, viruses, protozoans, Archaea, parasites, prions, fungi, and probably other undiscovered or unidentified organisms. By number of cells, the human cells of our body are outnumbered ten to one by the over one hundred trillion microbes living on and within the average human. If instead of cell population the comparison were based on genes that can be expressed and control biological functions, the human genes are outnumber one hundred to one. In addition to the gut microbiome, there are unique microbiomes on all aspects of the human body exposed to the external environment. Research activities are studying all areas of the human microbiome including, skin, oral, nasal, genitourinary, etcetera. The research findings to date are so dramatic that many scientists describe the microbiome as if a new major organ system of the body has just been discovered.

The organisms that make up the gut flora are a major source of the intestinal gasses produced during digestion and fermentation. The interaction between these organisms, food, and the human gut and brain are just beginning to be uncovered. More important than their major contribution to intestinal gas is their even more important contribution to human health and vitality.

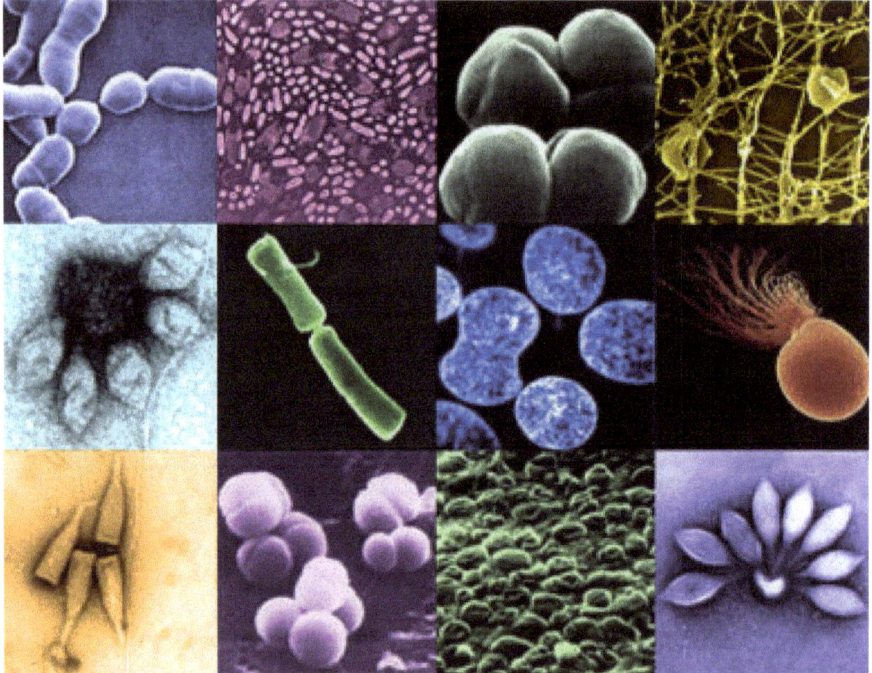

The human gut microbiome is made up of hundreds of trillions of organisms including Archaea, bacteria, parasites, prions, protists and viruses. They produce gasses such as hydrogen and methane that are constituents of intestinal gas.

The brain gut axis has been recognized for over a century. It has also been well recognized that information and influence travels in both directions. The brain can trigger digestive system symptoms and disorders including the common functional conditions such as irritable bowel syndrome. Digestive disorders frequently send signals to the brain and may lead to systemic anxiety, fear, depression, and distress. The brain central and autonomic nervous systems are intimately connected with the enteric nervous system of the gastrointestinal tract.

Gut intuition, know it in your gut, gut wrenching experience, gut wrong, gut check, butterflies in the stomach, gut instinct, gut reaction, listen to your gut, go with your gut, are all common expressions to describe the common experiences of intuition most commonly known as gut feelings. The gastrointestinal tract is sensitive to stress and emotion. Anger, anxiety, sadness, fear, elation are all among the many feelings that can trigger symptoms in the gut ranging from mild spasm to intense nausea, vomiting, cramps, diarrhea, and fecal incontinence.

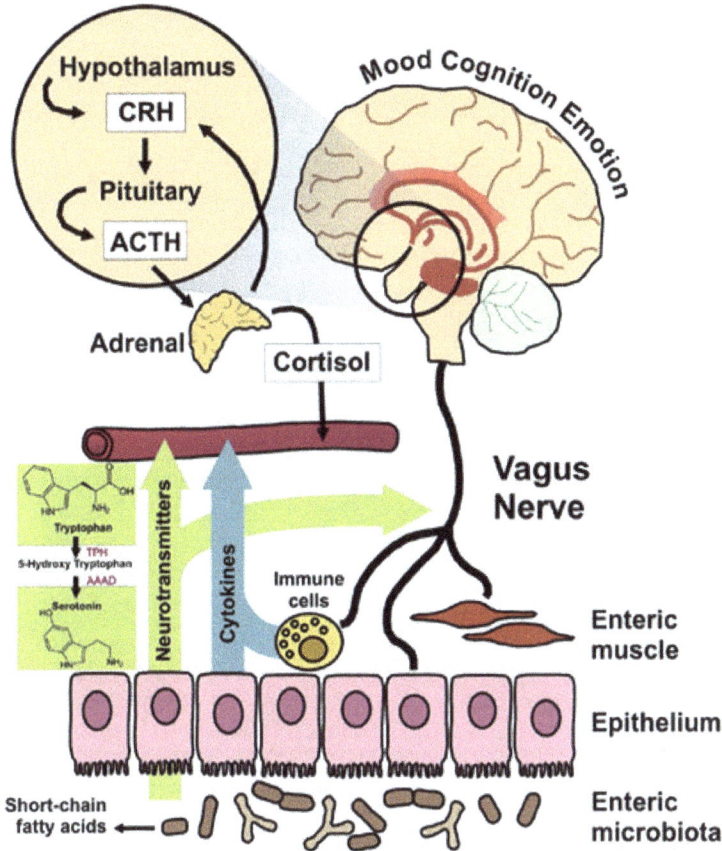

c431376.r76.cf2.rackcdn.com Creative Commons License

The brain has a direct effect on the digestive tract. As demonstrated by Ivan Pavlov, dogs accustomed to hearing a bell before being fed begin to salivate with just the sound of the bell even if no food is offered. The release of saliva, digestive enzymes, hormones, and gut motility can all be stimulated by thoughts generated by the brain alone.

Ninety-five percent of the body's supply of the well-recognized and critically important neurotransmitter serotonin is found in the gut. The brain and its serotonin receptors, representing only five percent of the body's serotonin, is a frequent target of prescription medications such as Prozac (fluoxetine). These pharmaceuticals are known as a selective serotonin re-uptake inhibitor (SSRI). The gut and the brain each have fifty percent of another important neurotransmitter, dopamine.

Gut Fermentation Syndrome

Gut fermentation syndrome is also known as the auto-brewery syndrome and is a rare medical condition in which not only gas but alcohol is produced within the gastrointestinal tract through endogenous fermentation. The alcohol produced is absorbed and can lead to intoxication if sufficient substrate is ingested into the digestive system. Numerous cases have been documented in the medical literature with isolation of the fermenting organism *Saccharomyces cerevisiae*. Interestingly enough many people use *Saccharomyces* and Brewer's yeast as a probiotic supplement. It has also been investigated, but eliminated, as a possible cause of sudden infant death syndrome.

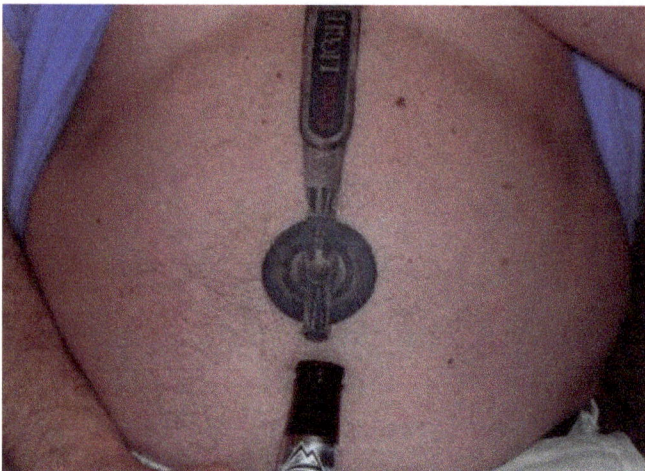

www.egotastic.com Creative Commons License

Claims of endogenous fermentation of this type have also been used as a defense against drunk driving charges. Often the defendant is required to submit to medical isolation and documentation that their blood alcohol level will rise spontaneously if given a fermentable carbohydrate rich meal. If the blood levels do not confirm the existence of the extremely rare disorder they are convicted of the driving while intoxicated charge and have additional medical expenses added to their penalty.

Alcoholic beverages, typically containing <1% to 40% ethanol by volume, have been produced and consumed by humans since pre-historic times. Ethanol is obtained fermentation using glucose that is produced from the hydrolysis of starch in the presence of yeast. Several of the benign bacteria in the intestine use fermentation as a form of anaerobic metabolism, which produces ethanol as a waste product. Human bodies contain some quantity of alcohol produced by these bacteria. In rare cases, this can be sufficient to cause "auto-brewery syndrome" in which intoxicating quantities of alcohol are produced by the bacterial flora of the gastrointestinal tract. Ethanol is further metabolized by the liver.

To 'Air' is Human Volume Two

High Altitude Living (see Atmospheric Pressure, Ideal Gas Laws)

The majority of the world's population lives close to the seashore and have the standard atmospheric pressure of one atmosphere found at sea level. A significant percentage of the world's population lives at higher altitudes with atmospheric pressures less than one atmosphere. One hundred and forty million people live at altitudes above 2,500 meters (8,200 ft.). M The higher above sea level you are, the lower is the atmospheric pressure you are subjected to. As a consequence, although the number of molecules of gas produced is identical, it will require a larger volume of space to contain it.

Those who travel to higher altitudes, whether by climbing a mountain, driving up a mountain road, or traveling by air, experience an increase in flatulence. The underlying principle is the same, according to the gas laws of physics a reduction in atmospheric pressure results in an increase in the volume of intestinal gas. Those who reside in high altitude communities become used to this degree of flatulence as normal for their elevation.

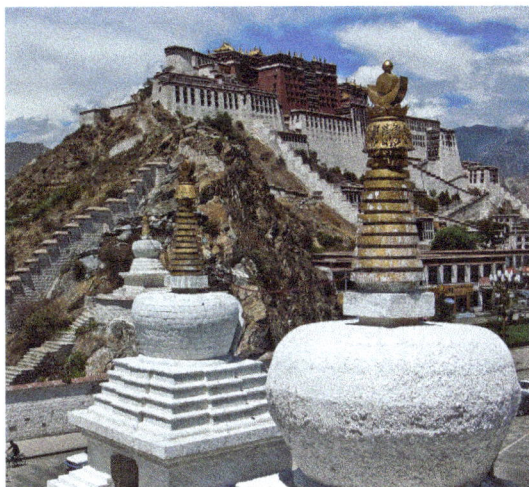

The Potala Palace, Lhasa, Tibet is higher yet at 11,450 feet altitude. Photo by Antoine Taveneaux
Creative Commons License

If you live in Denver Colorado, the mile high city with an elevation of five thousand one hundred and eighty three feet (one thousand six hundred and nine meters) feet above sea level, the volume will be larger than residing in Los Angeles or New York City. It is all relative as residing in Mexico City, which is at seven thousand three hundred and fifty feet (two thousand two hundred and forty meters), will produce a much larger volume than Denver. Working or living in high-rise buildings may also give rise to changes in atmospheric pressure. This is most readily demonstrated by taking a high-speed elevator in a high-rise building. The rapid decrease in atmospheric pressure traveling from the lower to the higher floors often results in pressure changes on the eardrum (tympanic membrane). The equalization of pressure on both sides of the tympanic membrane may give rise to an ear popping sensation.

Another important consideration for those engaged in high altitude activities is the recognition that the oxygen content of air decreases with an increase in altitude. The percentage saturation of hemoglobin with oxygen determines the oxygen content of the blood. Atmospheric pressure decreases exponentially with altitude, so while the O_2 fraction remains relatively constant the absolute amount of oxygen in a given volume of air decreases exponentially as well. At an altitude around 2,100 m (7,000 feet) above sea level, the oxygen saturation of hemoglobin begins to decrease dramatically.

Many air travelers are under the false impression that pressurization of the aircraft means the oxygen content of the air is the same as that on the ground at sea level. The aircraft is typically pressurized to maintain a cabin pressure equivalent to an altitude of approximately eight thousand feet. This leads to a reduction in the oxygen content of the air on the aircraft. Some normal individuals find this reduction in oxygen uncomfortable and develop headaches and other symptoms. Others are more sensitive, or recognize that their underlying medical condition requires that they have access to supplemental oxygen for their safe travel.

At an altitude of 5,000 m (16,000 ft.), the altitude of the Mount Everest base camp, hemoglobin oxygen saturation is reduced by fifty per cent. At the and only a third at the summit of Mount Everest at an altitude of 8,848 m (29,029 ft.) above sea level the oxygen saturation is reduced by two thirds. Travel to high altitude regions can lead to medical problems, from the mild symptoms of acute mountain sickness to life threatening high altitude pulmonary edema and cerebral edema. The higher the altitude, the greater the risk. For those with underlying circulatory or lung conditions the additional stress of even mildly lower oxygen content of the air can be potentially life threatening. Altitude sickness can develop rapidly and is a life-threatening condition requiring an immediate descent in altitude.

Hydrogen

Hydrogen and methane are two explosive gasses produced by the gut microbes. Their presence in farts make the fart ignitable and flammable, used to the amusement of some and the chagrin and painful burns of others. These same microorganisms continue their gas production in the feces after it exits the host digestive tract. Both hydrogen and methane are odorless. Hydrogen sulfide and other aromatic and volatile substances are also produced by the microorganisms in feces that produces its characteristic odor.

Hydrogen is lighter than air and lighter than helium. Unfortunately it is also explosively flammable. Hydrogen fires are less destructive to immediate surroundings because of the buoyancy of H_2, which causes heat of combustion to be released upwards as it ascends in the atmosphere. On May 6, 1937, the hydrogen filled German airship Hindenburg burst into flames while attempting to land at Lakehurst, New Jersey. In little more than 30 seconds, the largest object ever to soar through the air was incinerated.

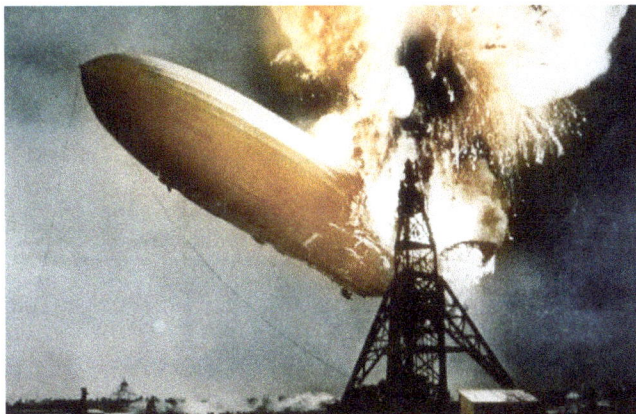

Public Domain

Hydrogen is a chemical element the symbol H and atomic number 1. It is the lightest element and in its single atom form it is by far the most abundant element in the universe, comprising approximately 75% of its total mass. In the earth's atmosphere as the diatomic H_2 molecule it is a colorless, odorless, tasteless, non-toxic, highly explosive gas. Most of the hydrogen on Earth is in molecules such as water and organic compounds because hydrogen readily forms covalent bonds. In 1766 Henry Cavendish was the first to identify hydrogen gas. In 1783 Antoine Lavoisier gave the element the name hydrogen (Greek ὕδρω hydro water and γενῆς genes creator) when he and Laplace confirmed Cavendish's finding that water is produced when hydrogen is burned.

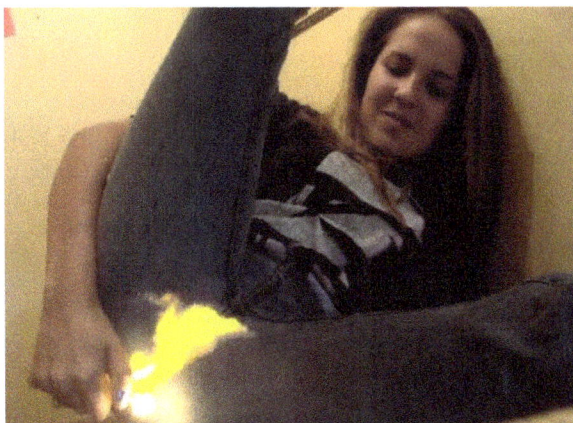

Moment of ignition of a fart, video is at youtu.be/Zt9rvaijpPY

Hydrogen and methane are the two flammable gasses that may be found in a fart making them flammable. Lighting a fart to see if one produces these gasses is actually a dangerous activity. Significant burns to the anogenital area have occurred as a result, especially when ignited without a clothing barrier. The popular television show *Mythbusters* filmed an episode confirming that many farts are indeed flammable. It appears that the network found the episode too provocative, and perhaps for liability concerns that children watching might attempt their own demonstrations decided to not 'air' the episode.

 Hydrogen, The Big Bang

For those entertained by the lighting of the hydrogen or methane of farts, there is another 'big bang' associated with hydrogen gas. According to the Big Bang theory of the origin of the universe, atoms were created as the super-heated and compressed dense mass of the universe expanded and cooled. It is virtually beyond our ability to comprehend the astronomical numbers of atoms in the universe. All the more remarkable is that after billions of years the cooling and expansion continues yet 90% plus of the energy and matter in the universe remains invisible to our scientific instruments and exploration to date.

Through the process of nuclear fusion within stars two atoms of hydrogen combined into one atom of helium. The process of fusion continued to create the heavier elements through stars and supernova. In spite of the billions of years that have passed since the Big Bang the development of the heavier elements is still in its infancy. 98% of all known matter in the universe is the simplest element hydrogen. Another 1% is the next earliest element helium. All of the other elements that populate our universe and that were created from stardust are less than 1% of the known elements.

The known universe is 99% hydrogen and helium, the two lightest elements and nearly always found as gases. Planets are the extreme oddity of being comprised of heaver elements of liquids and solids as well as gasses. Our planet Earth is a remarkable find with heavier elements as well as the primary element hydrogen. Most of the planets hydrogen has been oxidized in a ratio of two hydrogen atoms to one oxygen atom into $H2O$, liquid water, frozen ice, or water vapor depending on its local environment. The primary elements are gasses but as compounds they form other states of matter as liquids or solids. If you think of the human body we are primarily and predominantly hydrogen and oxygen gasses that have formed a liquid compound water.

When we observe an object with our vision what we are seeing are the photons of light energy being reflected back to us. The object is absorbing all of the wavelengths of light except those that are reflected back. So we are not actually seeing the object, what we are seeing is a reflection of what it did not absorb. Even though our reality may be an illusion, for the sake of our sanity I think it best to accept the illusion as reality and leave the details to the quantum physicists and scientists!

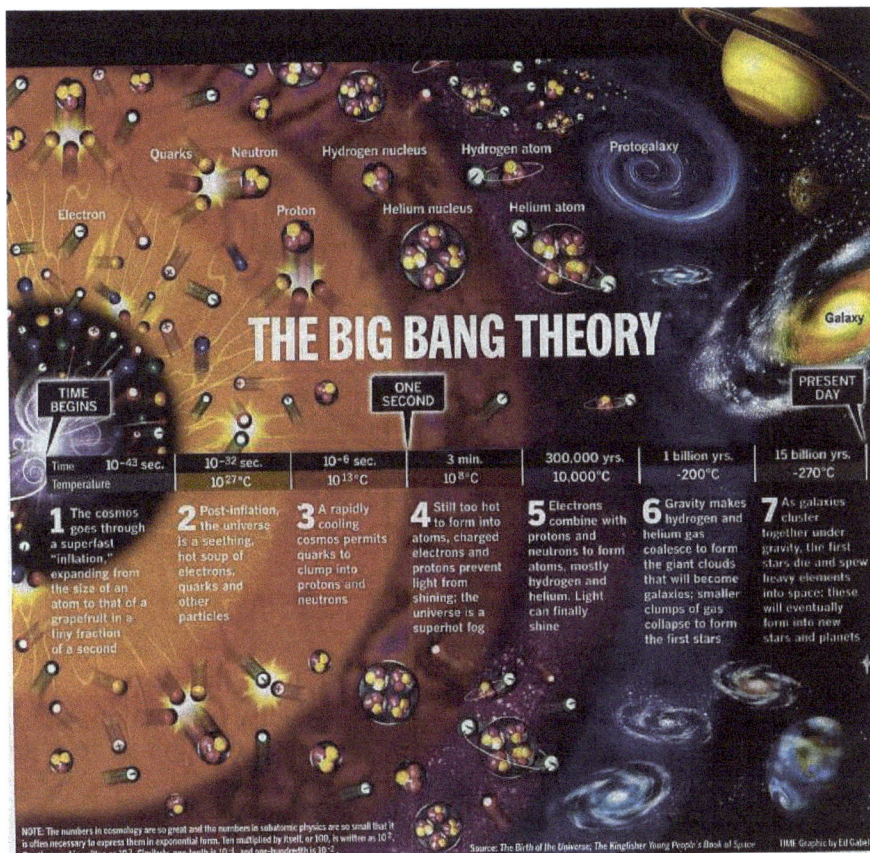

Big Bang Theory illustrated Time Magazine graphic

Hydrogen Sulfide

Hydrogen sulfide with the formula H_2S is a colorless gas with the characteristic foul odor of rotten eggs. It is heavier than air, poisonous, corrosive, flammable, and explosive and often results from the bacterial fermentation of organic material in anaerobic environments such as in swamps and sewers. H_2S also occurs in volcanic gases, natural gas, and well water.

Hydrogen sulfide (HS) is also produced by some cells and has biologically active signaling functions. Nitric oxide (NO) and carbon monoxide (CO) are the only other gases known to have this property. It acts as a relaxant of smooth muscle and as a vasodilator. It is also active in the brain where it may play a role in memory as well as Alzheimer's Disease, where the brains hydrogen sulfide concentration is markedly decreased. Hydrogen sulfide's ability to act as a vasodilator may be protective against cardiovascular disease. The sulfur group in allicin, garlic's bioactive component, is catabolized to hydrogen sulfide and may explain garlics reported cardio protective properties. Like nitric oxide, hydrogen sulfide is involved in the relaxation of the smooth muscle that causes vasodilation and erection of the penis. Nitric oxide and hydrogen sulfide appear to work via different mechanisms suggesting that new therapeutic options for erectile dysfunction and a variety of medical conditions may be possible.

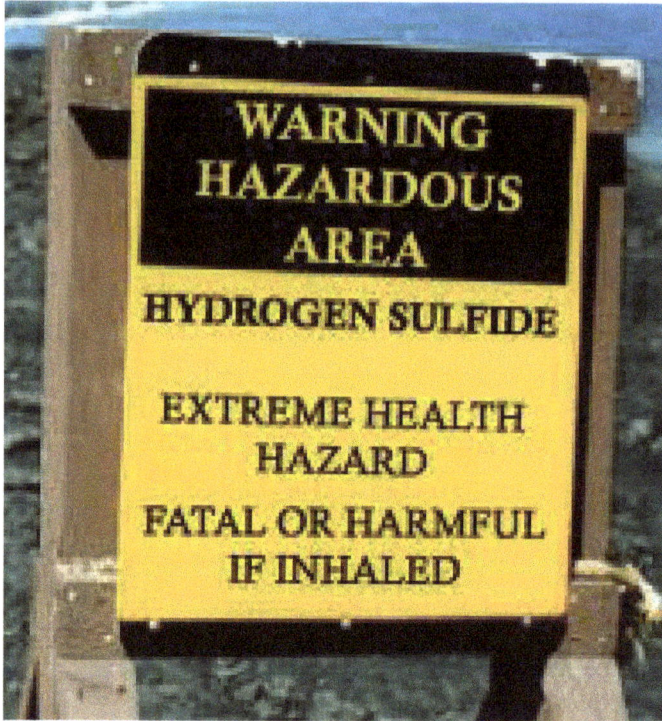

Public Domain

An excess of hydrogen sulfide can also be detrimental. The overproduction of HS is involved in the pathogenesis of type 1 diabetes and leads to the injury and death of the insulin producing beta cells. The injurious effects of Hydrogen sulfide have been implicated in mass extinctions that have occurred in the Earth's past. Buildup of hydrogen sulfide in the atmosphere, perhaps from major volcanic eruptions, may have caused the Permian-Triassic extinction event 252 million years ago.

Hydrogen Sulfide is found in high concentrations in the calderas of volcanoes, which is also where significant mining activity for sulfur takes place. In spite of the harsh conditions and dangerous gasses active mining for sulfur takes place in the crater of Kawah Ijen volcano in Java, Indonesia. Next to a sulfuric acid lake with a measured pH as low as 0.5 a number of vents in the caldera emit volcanic gasses like sulfur dioxide (SO_2) and hydrogen sulfide (H_2S). These gasses are channeled through ceramic pipes where the gasses are condensed into liquid sulfur as the gas cools. Deep red molten sulfur pours out of the pipes, further cools to the yellow mineral, which forms solid yellow cakes of sulfur, and are ten carried out of the area by miners in baskets. The miners work without protective equipment and have to hike up and down out of the high altitude volcanoes caldera twice a day. Typical miners earn the equivalent of $13 U.S. per day.

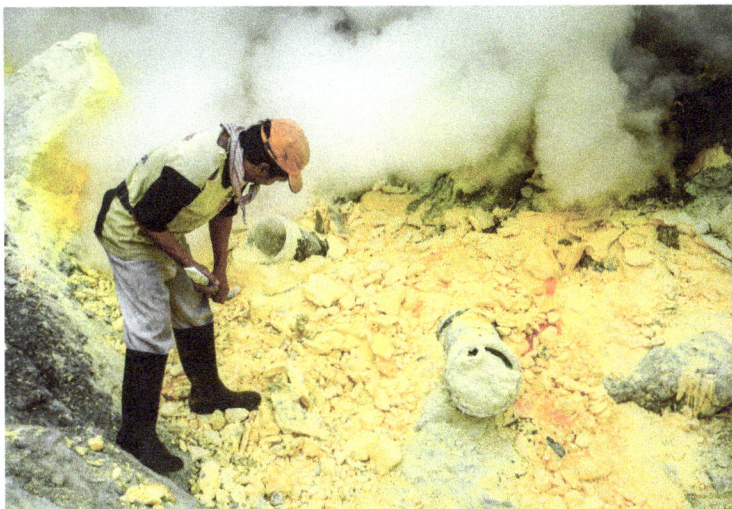

Sulfur mine. shutterstock/Zephyr_p

A number of Archaea organisms utilize hydrogen sulfide, and even elemental sulfur as an energy source. The relatively recent discovery of Archaea, and the organisms that are considered extremophiles, has revolutionized our understanding of life itself. These organisms can exist, and thrive in environments previously considered incompatible with life.

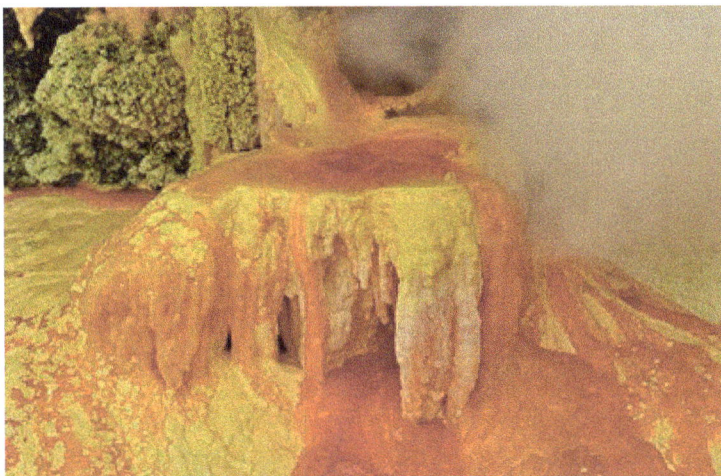

Olivier Grunewald.

Stanley Miller and Harold Urey became famous for their pioneering studies of what the early earth's atmosphere was like and what might have been brewing there millions of years ago. Using discharges of electricity as a substitute for lightning they used a few basic chemicals, water, methane, hydrogen and ammonia, to simulate the atmospheric conditions on Earth before life began. They demonstrated that some of the early building blocks of life were spontaneously created in this environment. Early experiments showed five to ten different amino acids, the building blocks for plants, animals, and fungi were generated.

Creative Commons License

In 1958 they added hydrogen sulfide to the mix and the long forgotten vials from their primordial-soup-in-a-bottle experiments were rediscovered just a few years ago. Using much more sophisticated analysis than was available over fifty years ago shows that the volcanic activity seeping hydrogen sulfide helped create the rich environment from which early life evolved. The recent analysis showed that by adding hydrogen sulfide the number of amino acids generated increased up to 23, with additional compounds and amines generated as well. Included in the new amino acids was methionine, which is a required building block for many life forms

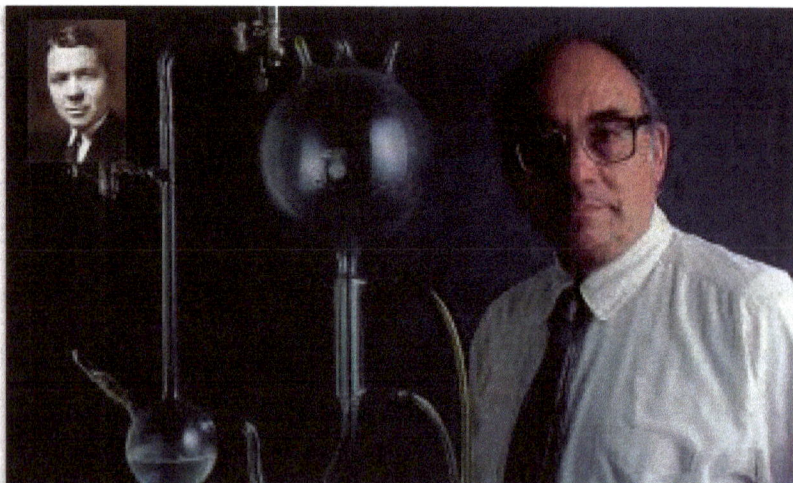

Harold Urey (inset) and Stanley Miller devised an experiment that revealed the earliest building blocks of life may have been generated in early planetary atmosphere of the Earth. Creative Commons License

Ideal Gas Law

Many aspects of the human body that deal with gasses, in particular the respiratory system and the gastrointestinal systems both deal with large volumes of gas. Unlike solids and liquids the gasses in nature are dramatically impacted by changes in temperature, pressure and volume. For example when the temperature of a gas increases its volume increases or if its volume cannot increase because it is contained than its pressure increases. The individual laws of physics discovered and named after Avogadro, Boyle, Charles & Gay-Lussac dealing with gas at different temperature, volume, and pressure have been combined into the ideal gas law: PV = nRT. The symbols represent the properties of the gas, P is pressure, V is volume, n is the amount in moles, R is the ideal gas law constant and T is temperature.

Ideal Gas Law

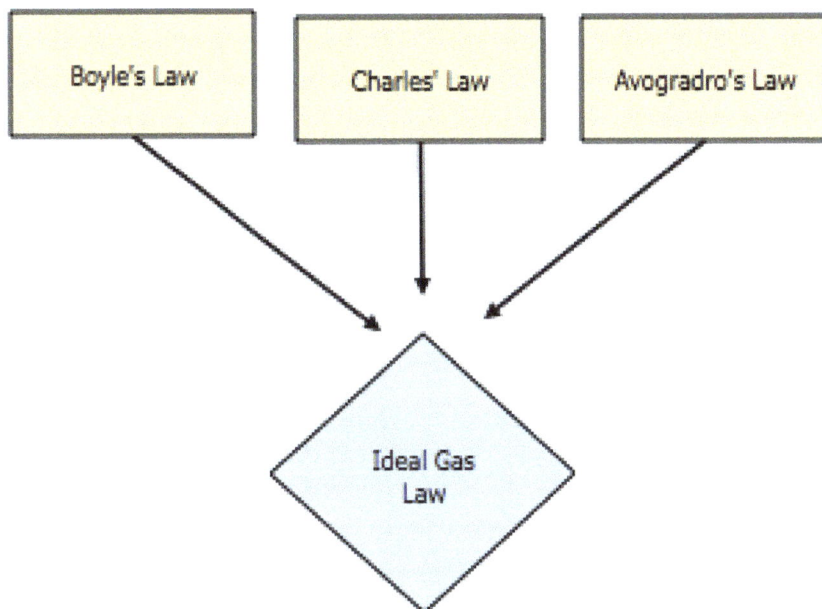

http://chemwiki.ucdavis.edu Creative Commons License

Farts are no exception and obey the ideal gas laws. The volume of a fart is related to its temperature and pressure. As an example, if you happen to have a fever and your body temperature is elevated the pocket of gas in your intestines will expand or the pressure will increase, or you will release a fart with more power volume and sound than usual. The laws of physics are the basis for the changing behavior of intestinal gas in scuba diving, mountain climbing, airplanes, and a wide variety of situations you may or may not have thought about.

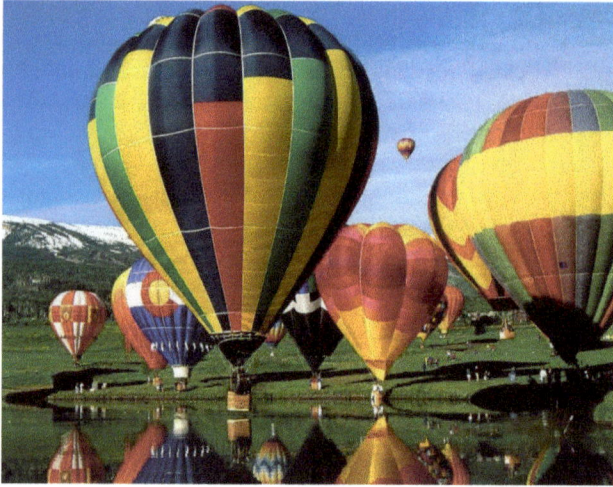

Hot air balloons are an example of hotter temperature leading to volume expansion. Creative Commons License.

Intestinal Gas, Therapy

When it comes to therapy for intestinal gas the first attempt is to identify foods or products that exacerbated, and avoid them. One can try an elimination diet, where one food or food group at a time our abstained from. If there is no improvement in the degree or symptoms related to intestinal gas a different food or food group is substituted for an elimination period.

One of the most common foods to which people are sensitive, which results in excess of gaseousness, is lactose intolerance. Lactose is the complex sugar found in milk and requires the enzyme lactase for its conversion to the two simple sugars, glucose and galactose, to allow its absorption. Most individuals have some degree of lactose intolerance, and can adequately digest small amounts of dairy product without symptoms. The symptoms of lactose intolerance become manifest when the amount of lactose consumed exceeds the individual's ability to produce lactase. The ability of the digestive track cells of the villi to produce lactase diminishes with age especially after infancy and childhood.

The avoidance of dairy products particularly in excess of the individual's lactase production results in symptom resolution. The most common symptoms are those of excessive gaseousness including distension and flatulence, and diarrhea. There are many dairy substitute products in the marketplace including those manufactured from rice, soy, various nuts such as almonds and cashews, coconuts, and others. Another approach is the commercial availability of the enzyme lactase itself. It may have already been added to the dairy product and is commonly found in the marketplace. Lactase supplements, which are taken orally with dairy products, are also available and effective.

To 'Air' is Human Volume Two

Another common source of excessive gaseous and this is a diet high in legumes and cruciferous vegetables. A number of vegetables have a high content of complex sugars known as raffinose, verbascose, and stachyose. The enzyme required to metabolize and digest these complex sugars is known as alpha-galactosidase. Humans as well as other animals do not have this enzyme, which is found only in plants. When the undigested complex sugar reaches the gut flora we microbes ferment and metabolize it releasing gases in the process. One approach is to reduce the quantity of these food products in the diet. In the case of beans soaking them for several hours, and in particular and allowing them to sprout, starts the process of alpha-galactosidase production within the bean itself. A simpler approach is taking an alpha-galactosidase supplement such as beano just prior to the meal. Alpha-Galactosidase is destroyed by heating, and that should not be added to foods prior to cooking or preparation.

Other food sensitivities such as to gluten are controversial. There is a known condition of gluten sensitive enteropathy also known as celiac disease, sprue, and nontropical sprue. In this condition a portion of the gluten known as gliadin damages the villi of the intestinal tract. As the damage continues the villi are blunted and shortened, eventually resulting in malabsorption. The inability to digest and process foods provides material for they gut microbiome to metabolize and release gases as well as causing diarrhea. A much larger portion of the population has reported sensitivity to gluten, and indeed a significant number do have difficulty digesting wheat and the other cereal grains that do contain gluten including rye, barley, and oats.

The sugar fructose most commonly found in fruits is a frequent source of intestinal gas and diarrhea if consumed in excess. All humans have a limited capacity to process the fruit sugar fructose. Nonnutritive sugars such as mannitol sorbitol and other food additives such as polysorbate-80 may cause excessive gaseousness as well. The most common foods related to belching and burping, known as eructation, are those, which contain gases in dilution such as carbonated beverages, beer, and champagne. Many foods also have very high air content. This includes whipped foods, baked goods including bread, fruit, ice cream, and others.

Some individuals are also prone to aerophagia. Everyone swallows air but those prone to aerophagia gulp down more than the average amount of air. The activities that can result in excess of aerophagia include rapid eating, drinking with the strong or from a bottle, tilting the head and neck back while swallowing, poorly fitting dentures, chewing gum or tobacco products, sucking or chewing on hard candies, as well as smoking. Talking while eating will also result in excessive swallowing. Individuals with sinus condition or postnasal drip tend to swallow their secretions frequently, every swallow also including about one teaspoonful of air.

Most of the individuals who have excessive burping and belching also have a hiatal hernia and gastroesophageal reflux disease GERD. In this condition the most common problem is inappropriate relaxation of the lower esophageal sphincter, when it should be closed tight after each swallow to prevent regurgitation. The gastric contents are usually very acidic from the addition of hydrochloric acid produced by the gastric glands. When this acidic material is refluxed into the esophagus irritation and damage of the esophageal lining may occur. If it occurs on a chronic basis the development of a change in the mucosal lining, known as a Barrett esophagus, may arise with an increased risk of the development of esophageal cancer.

The usual treatment for gastroesophageal reflux disease includes conservative measures such as reducing excess weight above normal, avoidance of foods and social habits that relax the lower esophageal sphincter. This includes fried foods, fatty foods, alcohol, tobacco, chocolate, and peppermint. Other measures may include elevating the head of the bed and avoiding any recumbent position until at least one hour after mealtime. Over-the-counter antacids and gastric acid suppressants are frequently used. If symptoms persist stronger prescription medication may be required to suppress the stomachs hydrochloric acid production. Fortunately, conservative treatment or acid suppressants are very effective. In some individuals the symptoms of heartburn is not present or minimal.

The gas symptomatology of bloating and distension is most frequently seen in irritable bowel syndrome. It is considered a functional gastrointestinal disorder most probably related to altered motility and heightened sensitivity to intraluminal pressure. Recent evidence suggests that alterations in the gut microbiome maybe playing a very important role in this condition. Some individuals benefit from introduction of the FODMAP dietary modification. Other conditions may also cause such symptoms including inflammatory bowel disease, bacterial infections, parasites, and others. One condition in particular that causes great concern in women is a possibility of ovarian cancer. This is typically a silent disease and bloating may be one of its first manifestations because of fluid buildup within the abdomen known as ascites.

Chronic pancreatitis and pancreatic insufficiency can result in enzyme deficiencies leading to malabsorption of fats, proteins, and carbohydrates. Fat malabsorption often leads to a form of diarrhea known as steatorrhea. In this condition the gas as well as the oily floating stool have the particularly characteristic offensive odor. Fortunately and pancreatic enzyme replacement supplements are commercially available and effective.

The approach to the intestinal gas problem of flatulence is addressed in the same manner as those above, as any unresolved burping, belching, and distension will nearly always eventually result in the gas passing down below. Because flatulence is of great social concern various treatment approaches have been attempted. One of the most important issues is to exclude significant underlying disease such as inflammatory bowel disease, bacterial overgrowth, parasites, and others.

Dietary modification or the usage of enzyme supplements can be very helpful. If this approach does not provide symptomatic improvement there are several over-the-counter safe products designed to be internal deodorants. The use of bismuth subgallate as well as chlorophyll products have been particularly successful. The use of pre-biotics, probiotics, and changes in the gut microbiome may be attempted. The use of antibiotics is usually limited to proven small intestinal bacterial overgrowth. Individuals who have undergone bariatric surgery, particularly with a gastric bypass, are especially prone to gas issues.

The use of activated charcoal has a long history of adsorbing toxins and gases. It has been used in chair cushions and other external modalities with some degree of effectiveness. Oral ingestion of activated charcoal has been less successful, presumably because the absorptive capacity of activated charcoal is markedly diminished by the time it reaches the colon. The addition of activated charcoal pads, as well as impregnating fabric with activated charcoal, the potential to provide a significant benefit. To be effective all of the gas released has to pass through activated charcoal. Formfitting underwear made with activated charcoal impregnated fabric has been very successful, albeit more expensive. The successful use of activated charcoal pads is dependent on the consumer placement of the pad in not allowing gas to escape. New product development including the use of other adsorbent material and metal ions hold promise for the availability of additional approaches.

As with all issues of health and wellness each person needs to be assessed individually. With the advances in the human genome project it is now recognized that it is not just the genetic blueprint in the DNA that makes up the individuals uniqueness. Although humans have approximately 23,000 genes these genes are also controlled by external factors in a process described as epigenetics. It is also now recognized that the human body is in essence more than just human cells. The human system includes the microbiome, the microorganisms that live on and within us. The gut-brain-microbiome-food axis demonstrates the intimate interconnectivity of these four elements. If one were to analyze the human system by the number of cells a human is comprised of approximately 10% human cells and 90% microbial cells. If one were to analyze the system on the basis of the number of genes, humans are approximately 1% human genes and 99% microbial jeans.

The era of personalized medicine will advance the understanding of both health and disease. The previous approach of using population-based medicine will be abandoned as technology and bioinformatics allows treatments to be specifically tailored to the individual's genome, microbiome, and metabolome. The effectiveness of therapy should increase dramatically along with a significant reduction in adverse reactions to medications. This approach will also avoid the time and monetary expense of medications that did not provide a benefit, even if fortunately they did not cause an adverse reaction. In the interval as these advances are being brought into clinical practice it remains the best approach to tailor the treatment plan to the individual. What works for one may not work for another. Until the science and technology sufficiently evolve it often takes a trial and error approach to find the best treatment approach for the individual. And it is the individual who can be the only judge if the treatment is successful or the search for a solution must continue.

Irritable Bowel Syndrome

Irritable bowel syndrome (IBS) also known as spastic colon is a functional disorder with the diagnosis based on symptoms of abdominal discomfort, bloating, and alteration of bowel habits. It may be predominated by diarrhea or constipation or alternation between the two. It is more common in women and symptoms can vary with the menstrual cycle. In the US there is an incidence of about 15% of the entire population. A diagnosis of irritable bowel syndrome is made on the basis of symptoms if celiac disease, lactose intolerance, parasites, and bacterial overgrowth have been excluded and there are no signs of weight loss, gastrointestinal blood loss, infections or family history of inflammatory bowel disease.

Irritable bowel syndrome occurs more commonly after an intestinal infection, or a stressful life event. A history of sexual abuse is found in thirty percent of women with irritable bowel syndrome. A serum test for anti-vinculin antibodies, which are elevated after intestinal infections is being investigated as a possible tool to identify irritable bowel syndrome. The cause of irritable bowel syndrome is unknown and there may be several different cause and conditions all pooled together under this diagnosis until further advances are made. The most popular theory is that IBS is a disorder of the complex neuroendocrine pathway between the brain and the gastrointestinal tract. Alternative approaches to the mind-body interactions have been proposed for irritable bowel syndrome and yoga, exercise, tai chi, meditation, and other modalities may offer benefits.

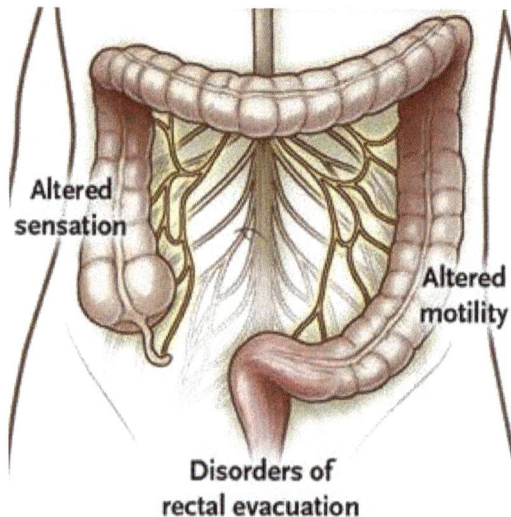

Altered
sensation

Altered
motility

Disorders of
rectal evacuation

blogs.nejm.org/now/wp Creative Commons License

Treatments have included dietary adjustments, medication and psychological interventions. FODMAP is an acronym that stands for Fermentable Oligosaccharides, Disaccharides, Monosaccharides, And Polyols. Restricting these short chain carbohydrates and related sugar alcohols, which are poorly absorbed in the small intestine. May be of benefit in irritable bowel syndrome. Many of these sugar alcohols including sorbitol, mannitol, xylitol, isomalt, and maltitol are added to commercial food products as non-nutritive bulk sweeteners. See entry on FODMAP diet for more details.

Newer prescription agents involving the neuroendocrine pathways, particularly serotonin agonist and antagonist are being studied. Other approaches using non-absorbable antibiotics such as rifaximin have provided relief for some patients, as has the use of probiotic agents to modulate the gut flora. Some believe the condition is triggered by changes in the gut flora and associated changes to the immune system. Fortunately irritable bowel syndrome is not associated with a higher risk if cancer or other conditions that would reduce life expectancy. It has a significant impact on quality of life and the economy. In the United States irritable bowel syndrome has been estimated to cost $10 billion a year in direct medical costs and an additional $20 billion in indirect costs.

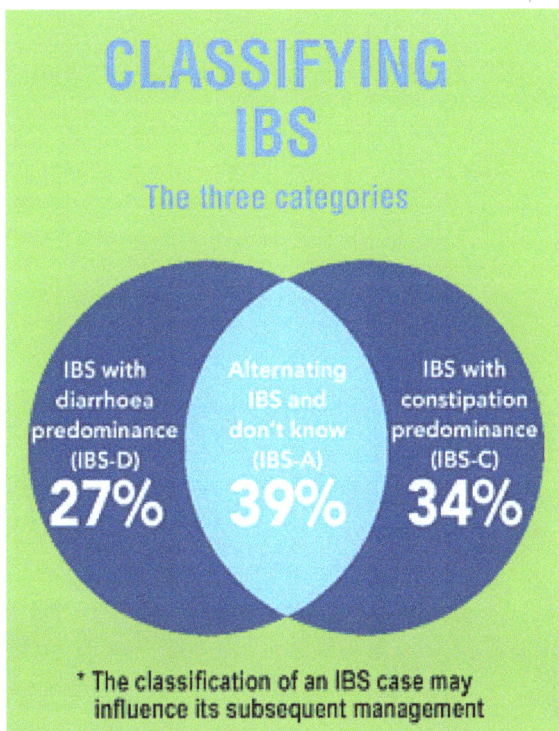

CLASSIFYING IBS
The three categories

IBS with diarrhoea predominance (IBS-D) **27%**

Alternating IBS and don't know (IBS-A) **39%**

IBS with constipation predominance (IBS-C) **34%**

* The classification of an IBS case may influence its subsequent management

media2.onsugar.com Creative Commons License

Lactase

Lactase is an enzymes involved in the hydrolysis of the disaccharide lactose into galactose and glucose. Lactase is located on the tips of microvilli along the lining of the small intestine. Levels of lactase decrease with weaning in a significant proportion of the human population. Other populations benefit from a mutation that is thought to have occurred over 5,000 years ago with the rise of the domestication of herd animals that allowed the continued ingestion of dairy products into adulthood. If the intake of lactose exceeds the availability of lactase to digest it the gut flora ferments the disaccharide. This gives rise to the symptoms of lactose intolerance, gas, cramps, and possibly diarrhea.

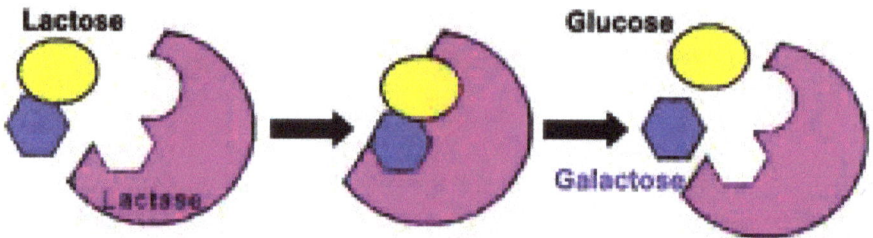

www.pharmaceutiucal-materials.com Creative Commons License

Lactose free foods are available where the lactase enzyme has already been added to the product to break down the lactose. The enzyme itself is also commercially available and should be taken with dairy products that contain lactose. Some dairy products, such as most hard cheeses, are lactose free on the basis of the production process. Acidophilus and Lactobacillus in yogurt and other foods also provides some lactase activity. Most people with lactose intolerance still have a nominal amount of the lactase enzyme and can digest lactose in very small quantities such as milk used as a creamer for coffee. Other dairy substitutes such as almond, rice, and soy 'milk' are lactose free.

Lactobacillus

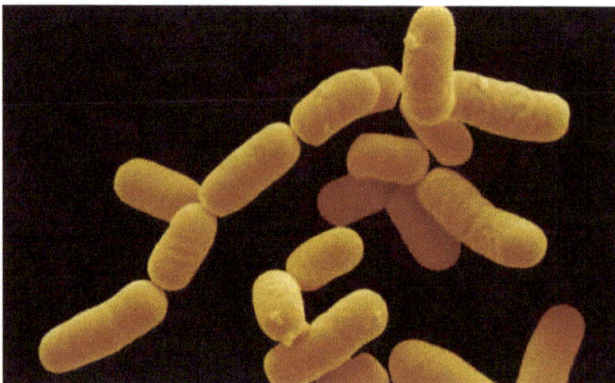

Lactobacillus rhamnosus, a probiotic bacterium www.theguardian.com Creative Commons License

Lactobacillus is a Gram-positive anaerobic rod-shaped bacterium that converts lactose and other sugars to lactic acid. The production of lactic acid makes its environment acidic which inhibits the growth of some harmful bacteria. In humans they are present in the vagina and the gastrointestinal tract where they make up a small portion of the gut flora. The genus Lactobacillus currently consists of over 180 species and encompasses a wide variety of organisms. Bifidobacterium was previously called *Lactobacillus bifidus* and has a separate entry under bifidobacterium.

Lactose

Lactose is a disaccharide of galactose and glucose that is found in milk from the Latin word lactis (milk). Lactose was discovered in milk in 1619 AD by Fabriccio Bartoletti. Varying between mammalian (the term derives from the distinctive characteristic of mammary glands). Lactose comprises between 2~8% of milk by weight. It is commercially extracted from whey, several million tons of which are produced annually as a by-product of the dairy industry. Whey is the liquid remaining after milk is curdled and strained, often for the production of cheese.

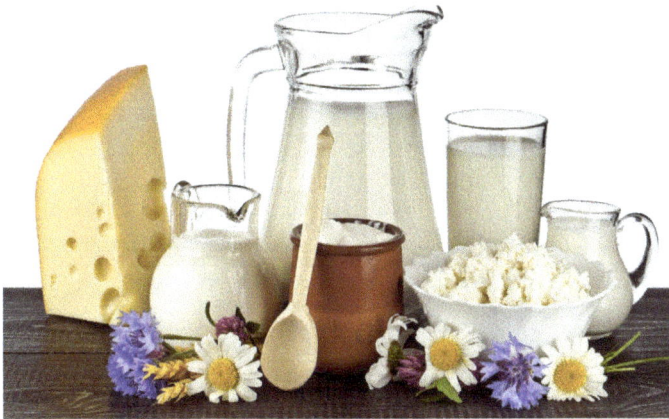

Dairy products. Creative Commons License

As a natural sugar found in milk and milk products it is found in cheese, ice cream, and processed foods, such as bread, cereal, and salad dressing. Hard cheeses typically have markedly reduced lactose content. Acidophilus milk and products that contain live Lactobacillus cultures such as in yogurts have reduced lactose content. Lactose free dairy products are also commercially available, as is the enzyme supplement lactase, which can be taken with the ingestion of lactose to help with its digestion, and processing.

Mammals nurse their infants on milk, which is rich in lactose. The villi of the small intestine secrete the enzyme lactase (β-D-galactosidase), which hydrolyses the lactose molecule into the simple sugars glucose, and galactose, which are easily absorbed. In most mammals the production of lactase decreases with the decreased consumption of reaching maturity.

Humans have continued to supplement their diet with milk from other mammals, especially those who developed herding practices of livestock, such as cattle, sheep, goats, camels, etc. The descendants of these populations appear to have induced the genetic tendency to maintain lactase production into adulthood. Other people have lost the ability to maintain significant lactase production and when the ingestion of lactose exceeds their enzymes capacity, the symptoms of lactose intolerance become apparent. When lactose is not digested by lactase the gut flora ferment it with the production of bloating, flatulence and occasional diarrhea from the osmotic properties if the sugar molecules drawing water into the digestive tract.

Any illness that damages the villi will result in a decrease if all of the enzymes and can aggravate underlying food intolerance. A viral or bacterial gastroenteritis, commonly referred to as a 'stomach flu or bug', will damage the villi and reduce the enzymes that would normally aid in digestion. The cell lining and villi of the small intestine tend to recover rapidly and thus for the few days following an infection dairy products are best avoided until the enzyme levels have recovered.

A major use of lactose is in the pharmaceutical industry where it is commonly used as inexpensive filler for pills because of its compressibility. It is also commonly used as inexpensive filler in a wide variety of food products. It is not unusual for individuals with known lactose intolerance to be unaware that they are ingesting sizable amounts of lactose in foods or pharmaceuticals. Reading the ingredient labels is important but the consumer has to be aware that lactose may be present if whey, whey protein, nonfat dry milk, milk sugar, powdered dairy product, etc. are included on the ingredient list. Unfortunately, lactose filler in pharmaceutical and nutraceutical products as well as nutritional and dietary supplements are rarely identified.

Lactose Intolerance

Lactose intolerance, also known as hypolactasia or lactase deficiency is the condition that arises when there is an insufficient quantity of the enzyme lactase, which is needed to metabolize the lactose commonly found in milk and dairy products. Hippocrates (460-370 BCE) was one of the first to recognize that many individuals had a difficult time digesting cow's milk. Lactase is an enzyme involved in the hydrolysis of the disaccharide lactose into galactose and glucose. Lactose intolerance is not an allergy and is not due to an immune response, it is due to the lack of a key digestive enzyme.

Lactase is located on the tips of microvilli along the lining of the small intestine. Levels of lactase decrease with weaning in a significant proportion of the human population. Other populations benefit from a mutation that is thought to have occurred over 5,000 years ago with the rise of the domestication of herd animals that allowed the continued ingestion of dairy products into adulthood. If the intake of lactose exceeds the availability of lactase to digest it the gut flora ferments the disaccharide. This gives rise to the symptoms of lactose intolerance, gas, cramps, and possibly diarrhea.

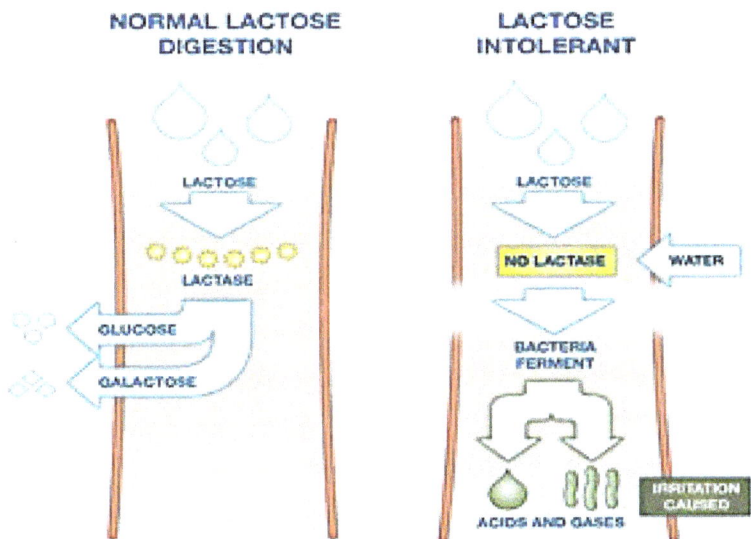

www.avonmorelactosefree.ie Creative Commons License

Lactose is a disaccharide of galactose and glucose that is found in milk from the Latin word lactis (milk). Lactose was discovered in milk in 1619 AD by Fabriccio Bartoletti. Varying between mammalian (the term derives from the distinctive characteristic of mammary glands). Lactose comprises between 2~8% of milk by weight. It is commercially extracted from whey, several million tons of which are produced annually as a by-product of the dairy industry. Whey is the liquid remaining after milk is curdled and strained, often for the production of cheese.

Mammals nurse their infants on milk, which is rich in lactose. The villi of the small intestine secrete the enzyme lactase (β-D-galactosidase), which hydrolyses the lactose molecule into the simple sugars glucose, and galactose, which are easily absorbed. In most mammals the production of lactase decreases with the decreased consumption of milk upon reaching maturity, a condition known as primary lactase deficiency. Secondary lactase deficiency arises when the intestinal villi are damaged, such as by gastroenteritis, celiac disease, parasites, etcetera. Congenital lactase deficiency is a very rare autosomal dominant inherited condition most often seen in the Finnish population. Certain populations, which developed dairy herds and persisted in milk consumption favored those who had a genetic variation now known as the lactase persistence allele. DNA evaluation of ancient skeletons revealed that this beneficial mutation developed in Europe and Russia over four thousand years ago. Seventy-five percent of African-American, Jewish, Native American, and Mexican American populations are lactose intolerant.

As a natural sugar found in milk and milk products it is found in cheese, ice cream, and processed foods, such as bread, cereal, and salad dressing. Hard cheeses typically have markedly reduced lactose content. Acidophilus milk and products that contain live Lactobacillus cultures such as in yogurts have reduced lactose content. Lactose free dairy products are also commercially available, as is the enzyme supplement lactase, which can be taken with the ingestion of lactose to help with its digestion, and processing.

Worldwide prevalence of lactose intolerance in recent populations (schematic)

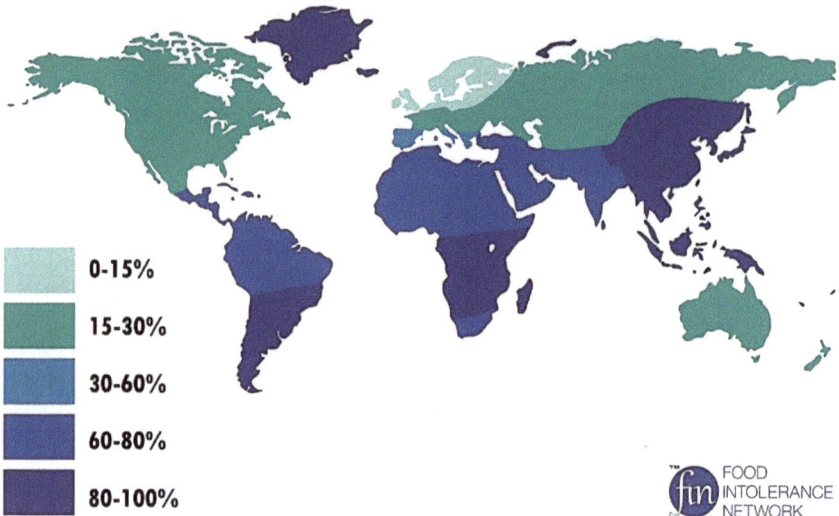

- 0-15%
- 15-30%
- 30-60%
- 60-80%
- 80-100%

FOOD INTOLERANCE NETWORK

upload.wikimedia.org/wikipedia/commons Author: NmiPortal Creative Commons License

Humans have continued to supplement their diet with milk from other mammals, especially those who developed herding practices of livestock, such as cattle, sheep, goats, camels, etc. The descendants of these populations appear to have induced the genetic tendency to maintain lactase production into adulthood. Other people have lost the ability to maintain significant lactase production and when the ingestion of lactose exceeds their enzymes capacity, the symptoms of lactose intolerance become apparent. When lactose is not digested by lactase the gut flora ferment it with the production of bloating, flatulence and occasional diarrhea from the osmotic properties if the sugar molecules drawing water into the digestive tract.

Any illness that damages the villi will result in a decrease if all of the enzymes and can aggravate underlying food intolerance. A viral or bacterial gastroenteritis, commonly referred to as a 'stomach flu or bug', will damage the villi and reduce the enzymes that would normally aid in digestion. The cell lining and villi of the small intestine tend to recover rapidly and thus for the few days following an infection dairy products are best avoided until the enzyme levels have recovered.

A major use of lactose is in the pharmaceutical industry where it is commonly used as inexpensive filler for pills because of its compressibility. It is also commonly used as inexpensive filler in a wide variety of food products. It is not unusual for individuals with known lactose intolerance to be unaware that they are ingesting sizable amounts of lactose in foods or pharmaceuticals. Reading the ingredient labels is important but the consumer has to be aware that lactose may be present if whey, whey protein, nonfat dry milk, milk sugar, powdered dairy product, etc. are included on the ingredient list. Unfortunately, lactose filler in pharmaceutical and nutraceutical products as well as nutritional and dietary supplements are rarely identified.

Dairy Product	Lactose (grams)	Dairy Product	Lactose (grams)
American Cheese, processed (1 slice, 1 oz)	1.17	Butter (1 tbsp)	0.01
Blue Cheese, crumbled (1/2 cup)	0.34	Sour Cream, cultured (1 tbsp)	0.02
Brie Cheese (1 oz)	0.13	Half and Half Creamer (1/2 cup)	0.19
Cheddar Cheese (1 oz)	0.15	Heavy Whipping Cream (1/2 cup)	0.07
Cottage Cheese, creamed, large curd (1/2 cup)	2.80	Milk: Fluid Whole, 2%, 1% (1 cup)	12.32
Cottage Cheese, creamed, small curd (1/2 cup)	3.00	Milk: Dry (1/4 cup)	12.29
Cream Cheese (1 tbsp)	0.32	Milk: Evaporated (1/2 cup)	12.65
Feta Cheese (1/2 cup)	3.07	Milk: Goat (1 cup)	10.85
Mozzarella Cheese, shredded (1/2 cup)	0.58	Milk: Human (1 cup)	16.95
Parmesan Cheese, hard (1 oz)	0.23	Milk: Lactaid (1 cup)	0.00
Provolone Cheese (1 oz)	0.16	Yogurt, Greek, plain (6 oz container)	5.51
Ricotta Cheese (1/2 cup)	0.33	Yogurt, plain, 8 grams protein (8 oz container)	10.58
Swiss Cheese (1 oz)	0.37	Yogurt, plain, 12 grams protein (8 oz container)	15.98

Source: USDA, ARS National Agricultural Library: Nutrient Data Laboratory
Amount of lactose may vary by brand. Read labels carefully.

Creative Commons License

Lactose free foods are available where the lactase enzyme has already been added to the product to break down the lactose. The enzyme itself is also commercially available and should be taken with dairy products that contain lactose. Some dairy products, such as most hard cheeses, are lactose free on the basis of the production process. Acidophilus and Lactobacillus in yogurt and other foods also provides some lactase activity. Most people with lactose intolerance still have a nominal amount of the lactase enzyme and can digest lactose in very small quantities such as milk used as a creamer for coffee. Other dairy substitutes such as almond, rice, and soy 'milk' are lactose free.

Le Pétomane

Joseph Pujol (1857 – 1945) was a stage performer from 1887 to 1914, and first performed on the Moulin Rouge stage in Paris in 1892. He had the unusual ability to inhale air into his colon through his anus and expel it at will. With the stage name Le Pétomane, French for the fart maniac, he was also affectionately known as 'the fartiste'.

With sufficient colonic inhalations and exhalations he was able to minimize the odor and control the sounds emanating from his anus to such a degree that he could play musical tunes. To assure that there was no odor he also underwent regular colonic irrigations before performances. Appearing on stage in red cape, white cravat, and black trousers, with a pair of white gloves held in the hands, he displayed the incongruous touch of elegance that added to his charm. A program of fart impressions followed, including contrasting the hearty fart of the miller with the timid fart of the young girl.

He proceeded to demonstrate the diffidence of the fart of the bride on her wedding night (almost inaudible) compared to the fart of the bride a week later (a lusty raspberry). His musical impersonations included an imitation of a tuba player on his instrument. He stunned the audience with a majestic ten-second fart, which he likened to a couturier cutting six feet of calico cloth. He would play *Le Marseilles* on his personal human wind instrument, his colon, even though he could only produce four notes do, mi, so, and the octave do. To add to his musical repertoire he would insert a tube offstage into his rectum and attach it to the musical instrument the ocarina. Then playing *O' Sole Mio* he would invite the audience to sing along.

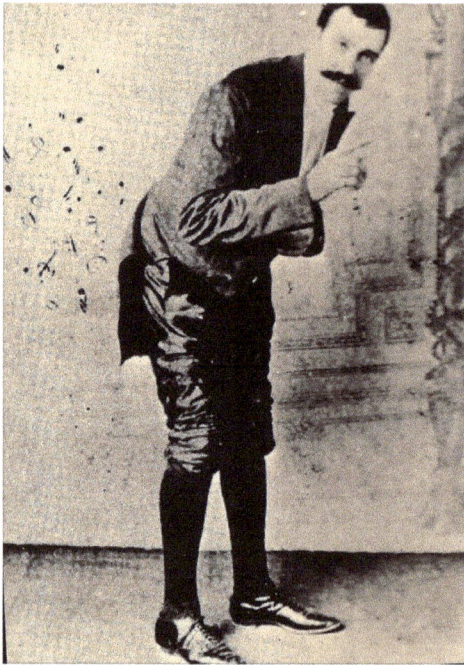

Joseph Pujol (Le Pétomane) 1857, Public Domain

Replacing the musical instrument at the end of the tube with a cigarette he used his colon to inhale. After withdrawal of the tube he would exhale the cigarette smoke out of his behind. For the grand finale he would imitate a twenty-one-gun salute, and the Great 1906 San Francisco earthquake with a thunderous roar that went on for over five continuous minutes. He would end his performance by blowing out a candle at a distance of three feet. Other than Harry Houdini, he was the highest paid stage performer in Europe and was earning a salary of twenty thousand francs per week. This was substantially more than the eight thousand francs per week salary of his contemporary Sarah Bernhardt who was considered the leading lady of the stage at that time. King Leopold II of Belgium and Edwards Prince of Wales came incognito to see Le Pétomane perform. Sigmund Freud attended a performance, and perhaps inspired, went on to describe his theory of anal fixation.

At one point he was embroiled in a disagreement with his stage manager and was going to perform in a different venue. The manager went to the courts and got a judicial injunction preventing Le Pétomane from performing elsewhere. During the court hearing Le Pétomane demonstrated his unique abilities in front of the court (he judge did not rule him out of order, or in contempt of court). Le Pétomane decided to offer his farting services and performance for free in a public display, but the manager and the court decision forbade him to fart in public.

When he died, the physicians of the day wanted to do a postmortem examination to find out how he had such remarkable anal control. The family held onto his body until enough decomposition set in that they no longer had to fear grave robbers retrieving the body for science. Joseph Pujol's memorable life lives on in the cinematic and stage arts. In Mel Brooks' 1974 movie Blazing Saddles, with many memorable fart scenes, there is an inside joke. It is an artistic acknowledgement to Joseph Pujol with Mel Brooks himself playing Governor William LePetomane.

Methane

Methane is produced in the human intestinal tract by microbial organisms. Methanogens are microorganisms of the Kingdom Archaea, not bacteria as previously thought. They produce methane as a metabolic byproduct in anaerobic conditions when oxygen is not present. Methanogens have been found in a variety of extreme environments and an thrive and reproduce in boiling water as well as in ice cores taken miles down in arctic glaciers. They are common in wetlands, where they produce marsh gas, and in the digestive tracts of animals and humans where they generate the methane content of flatulence as well as the ruminant belch. Higher methane concentrations in intestinal gas have been associated with decreased gastrointestinal tract motility and constipation.

Hydrogen and Methane are combustible gasses. In the presence of oxygen and an ignition source you have a potent flammable commodity. When methane burns it has a characteristic blue flame that you may see in a pilot light if you have a gas stove or furnace. Adolescent males and those who remain as adolescents intellectually have a fondness for demonstrating their dragon like ability to be human flamethrowers by igniting their farts. This is not a recommended activity and severe injury has resulted from successful attempts to ignite farts.

Hydrogen and methane are the two flammable gasses that may be found in a fart making them flammable. Lighting a fart to see if one produces these gasses is actually a dangerous activity. Significant burns to the anogenital area have occurred as a result, especially when ignited without a clothing barrier. The popular television show *Mythbusters* filmed an episode confirming that many farts are indeed flammable. It appears that the network found the episode too provocative, and perhaps for liability concerns that children watching might attempt their own demonstrations decided to not 'air' the episode.

On occasion dung and excrement can be more than just flammable, it can be explosive. The microorganism that produce hydrogen and methane that lead to ignitable farts continue their activity while sitting in a pile. For those foolish enough to light a match in a pile of cow dung to see what happens up close and personal the link to the video above should be convincing.

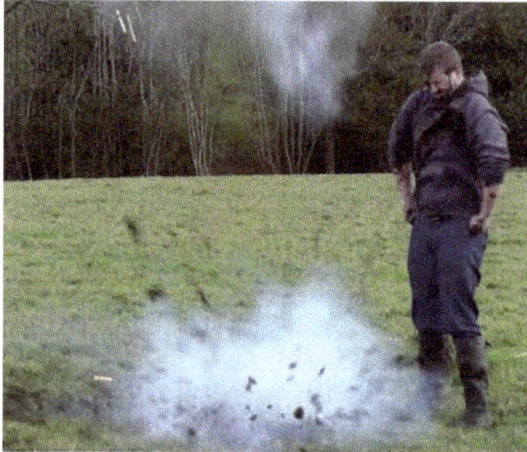

Lighting a match to a pile of cow dung is not a sign of higher intelligence. The methane and hydrogen generated by the microbes active in the dung pile may accumulate to explosive levels.
youtu.be/bZI1eeV88lQ

One of the more unusual injuries from a lit fart was second and third degree burns on the buttocks and a broken arm. The heavy gentlemen was sitting on the toilet defecating and farting extensively for a period of time. Being overweight his buttocks formed a firm seal around the toilet seat retaining all of the gasses in the enclosed space of the toilet bowl. He was smoking at the time and made a little space under his cheeks to innocently toss the lit cigarette into the toilet bowl. It promptly ignited blowing him off the seat, shattering the toilet bowl and causing extensive burn injuries to his buttocks. His wife called the paramedics and as he was being carried down the stairwell to the waiting ambulance he told them what caused the explosion. They laughed so hard they dropped the gurney thus breaking his arm.

Methane, Greenhouse Gases & Global Warming

'The primary greenhouse gases in the Earth's atmosphere are water vapor, carbon dioxide, methane, nitrous oxide, and ozone. Venus is a prime example of the planetary temperature consequences of the greenhouse effect. Nitrogen (N 2), oxygen (O 2), and argon (Ar), major components of the atmosphere are not greenhouse gases because they are minimally affected by infrared radiation. Clouds, composed of water droplets or ice crystals, do contribute to the greenhouse effect since they absorb and emit infrared radiation.

Water vapor accounts for about 50% of the Earth's greenhouse effect, with clouds contributing 25%, carbon dioxide 20%, and the minor greenhouse gases and aerosols accounting for the remaining 5%. Methane has a twenty fold greater impact on the greenhouse affect then carbon dioxide, when measured by weight. As a percentage however methane has a much smaller effect since it is found in relatively small amounts. The most important constituents of the greenhouse gasses are water vapor, clouds, carbon dioxide, methane, and ozone. Less important contributors include sulfur hexafluoride, hydro fluorocarbons, and per fluorocarbons.

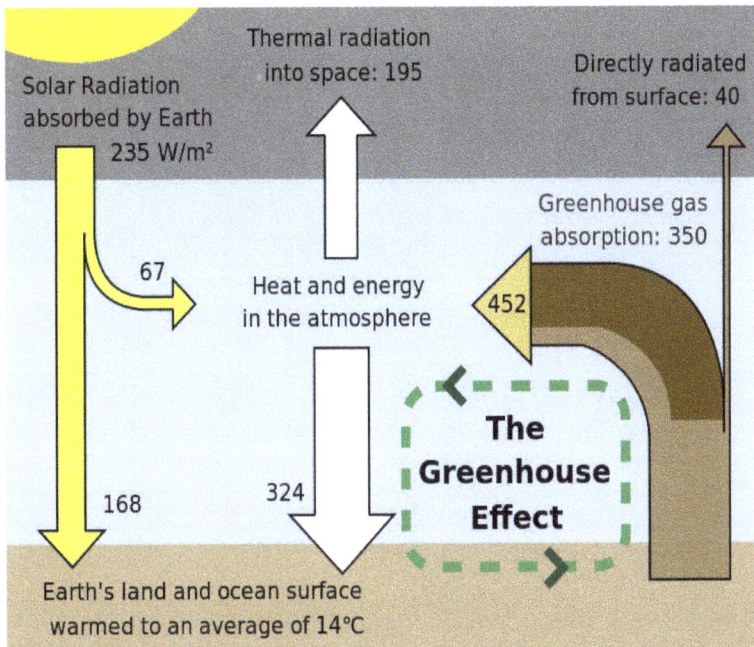

The figure shows the flows of energy between space, the atmosphere, and the Earth's surface, and how these flows trap heat near the surface and create the greenhouse effect. Energy exchanges are expressed in watts per square meter (W/m²). The sun is responsible for virtually all energy that reaches the Earth's surface. Of the surface heat captured by the atmosphere, more than 75% can be attributed to the action of greenhouse gases that absorb thermal radiation emitted by the Earth's surface. The atmosphere in turn transfers the energy it receives both into space (38%) and back to the Earth's surface (62%). The process by which energy is recycled in the atmosphere to warm the Earth's surface is known as the greenhouse effect. Creative Commons License

The atmospheric lifetime measures the time required to restore equilibrium in its concentration in the atmosphere. Water vapor has an atmospheric lifetime of approximately nine days in striking contrast to carbon dioxide of 30 years and N2O 114 years. The Earth's surface temperature is partly dependent on the balance between the absorption of radiant energy from the sun, and its reflection and re-radiation of energy back to space.

An earlier period of widespread glaciation (Snowball Earth) came to abrupt end about 550 MYA when a colossal volcanic outgassing raised the atmospheric CO2 concentration to 12%, about 350 present day levels. The extreme greenhouse conditions resulted in the deposition of calcium carbonate as limestone at the rate of over a foot each year. This brought a close to the Precambrian eon, and was succeeded by the warner Phanerozoic times with the appearance of multicellular animal and plant life. There has not been a recurrence of such a dramatic greenhouse effect since. No volcanic carbon dioxide emissions today are less than 1% of human production.

Based on measurements from Antarctic ice cores, the concentrations of carbon dioxide in the atmosphere are now 30% higher than levels before the industrial revolution. The levels had not changed appreciably in over 10,000 years. Although human activity only accounts for 5% of the greenhouse gasses, the naturally occurring amount was closely balanced by the Earths capacity to utilize the carbon sink of photosynthesis. Greenhouse gas production from human activity is mainly due to deforestation, the combustion of fossil fuels, livestock enteric fermentation and manure management, and landfill emissions. In terms of biomass bacteria would be the main contributors to global warming by their methane production. Other contenders nominated have been termites, which have over 2000 species and are prolific methane producers (initial reports suggested that they produce 40% of global methane), livestock such as cows, sheep, and pigs, and lastly dinosaurs, which are no longer around to defend their reputations.

A ruminant (Latin *ruminare* - to chew over again) is a mammal that digests plants in a multi compartment stomach through bacterial fermentation. It regurgitates the semi-digested mass, called cud, and chews it again and repeats the swallow. The process of re-chewing the cud is called "ruminating". There are about 150 species of ruminants, which include both domestic and wild species. Ruminating mammals include cattle, goats, sheep, giraffes, yaks, deer, camels, llamas, and antelope. Ruminant fermentation is a significant contributor to global methane production, which is over twenty times as potent greenhouse gas. Actually it is not the ruminant itself but the protist within its microbiome that generates hydrogen from the breakdown of cellulose. Within the protist is another organism Archaea, acting as a mutualist that converts the hydrogen to methane. To incentivize efforts to reduce livestock methane production a number of countries have proposed taxes on the release of greenhouse gasses. In spite of it being labeled as a flatulence tax, the predominant source of global warming from ruminants comes from fermentation in their multi compartment stomachs. It should really be called a burping and belching tax, but that is not as newsworthy.

Carbon dioxide, methane, nitrous oxide (N_2O) and three groups of fluorinated gases (sulfur hexafluoride (SF_6), hydro fluorocarbons (HFCs), and per fluorocarbons (PFCs)) are the major greenhouse gases impacted by human activity. These are regulated under the Kyoto Protocol an international treaty that was adopted in 2005. Nitrogen dioxide (NO_2) warms the atmosphere 310 times more than carbon dioxide and methane 21 times more than carbon dioxide. Although CFCs are greenhouse gases, regulations were initiated because CFCs' cause ozone depletion, not because of their contribution to global warming. Ozone depletion itself has a relatively minor effect on greenhouse warming.

Methane, Natural Gas

Natural gas is a naturally occurring mixture of hydrocarbon gases that consists primarily of methane. Smaller quantities of the higher alkanes such as ethane, propane, butanes, and pentanes are also often present. Other components that are commonly removed before marketing as a fuel can include hydrogen sulfide, carbon dioxide, water vapor, nitrogen, oxygen, and helium.

Natural gas is often used as an energy source for heating, cooking, and electricity generation. It is also used as fuel for vehicles and as a chemical feedstock in the manufacture of plastics and other commercially important organic chemicals. It contributes to less global warming as it produces 30 per cent less carbon dioxide than using petroleum and forty-five percent less than using coal as a fuel source.

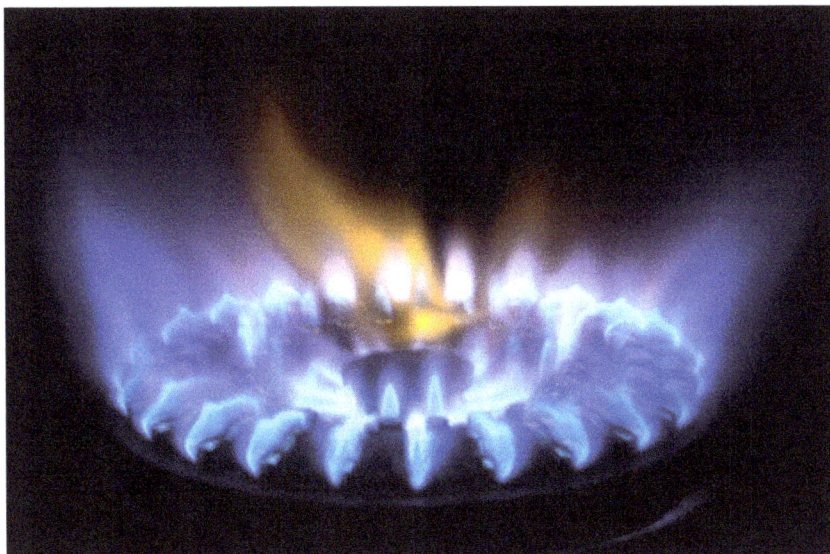

Creative Commons License

Natural gas is found in deep underground natural rock formations or associated with other hydrocarbon reservoirs in coal beds and as methane clathrates. Petroleum is also another resource found in proximity to and with natural gas. Most natural gas was created over time by two mechanisms: biogenic and thermogenic. Biogenic gas is created by methanogen organisms in marshes, bogs, landfills, and shallow sediments. Deeper in the earth, at greater temperature and pressure, thermogenic gas is created from buried organic material.

The location of shale gas compared to other types of gas deposits.

Shale gas in the United States is rapidly increasing as a source of natural gas. Led by new applications of hydraulic fracturing technology and horizontal drilling, development of new sources of shale gas has offset declines in production from conventional gas reservoirs, and has led to major increases in reserves of US natural gas. Large quantities of methane exist in the form of hydrates on offshore continental shelves and in the permafrost of the arctic regions. Hydrates are formed in the presence of a combination of high pressure and low temperature. Technology has yet to be developed yet to make the extraction economically viable.

Methane, Biogas

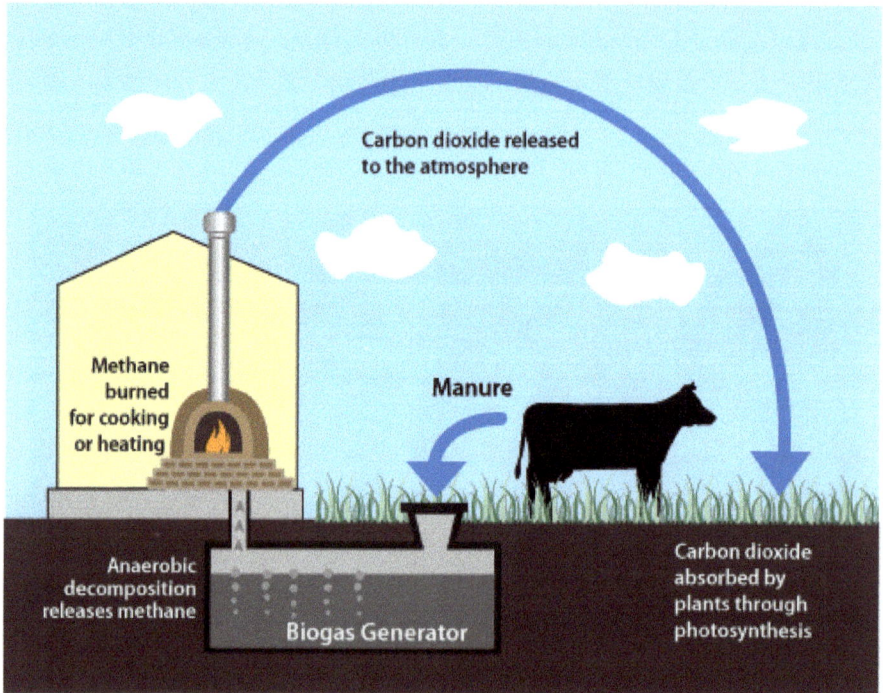

Carbon dioxide released to the atmosphere

Methane burned for cooking or heating

Manure

Anaerobic decomposition releases methane

Biogas Generator

Carbon dioxide absorbed by plants through photosynthesis

Creative Commons License

Biogas is produced by the anaerobic breakdown of organic biomass. The breakdown may require several different organisms acting in concert. For example the ruminant animal cannot digest cellulose without assistance from protist that reside in its gut microbiome. The protist generate hydrogen in the process of cellulose breakdown, which would be detrimental to the protist without the assistance of Archaea. The methanogenic Archaea actually reside within the protist and convert the hydrogen to methane. The sources of methane actually live in symbiotic relationships with other life, including termites, ruminants, and cultivated crops. When methane is produced with the decay of biomass it is referred to as biogas. Sources of biogas include swamps, marshes, landfills, manure, sewage sludge, and enteric fermentation.

Landfill gas has methane concentrations of approximately fifty percent. Waste treatment technologies can produce biogas of up to seventy-five percent methane. Biogas can be cleaned and upgraded to natural gas standards and is referred to as bio methane. One cow produces the manure in one day to generate three-kilowatt hours of electricity, enough to power a one hundred watt light bulb for twenty-four hours. If you imagine every cow having a one hundred watt light bulb illuminated from its digestive tract end product, you would have a new definition of a taillight.

 Methane, Dinosaurs

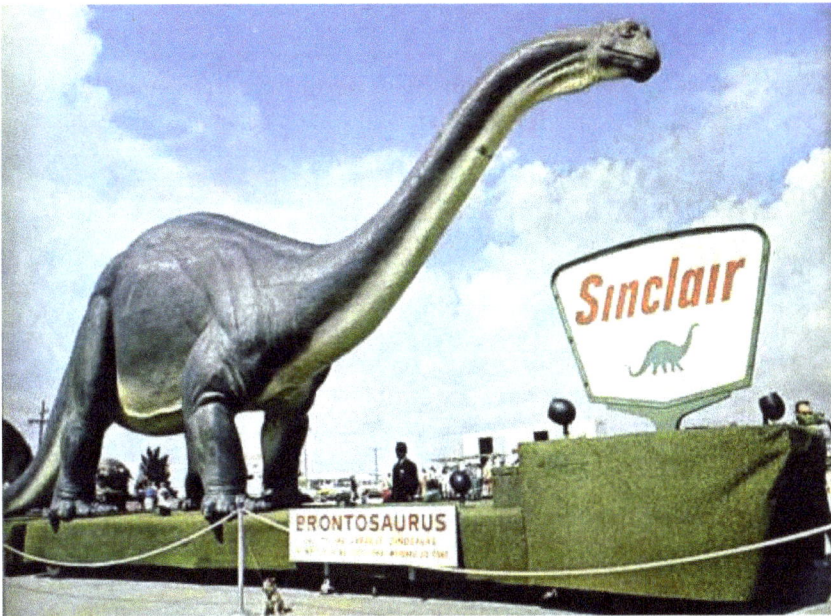

American Oil & Gas Historical Society

In 1933, the Sinclair Oil Corporation had an exhibit at the World's Fair in Chicago, suggesting that the world's oil reserves were created from material from the dinosaurs of the Mesozoic Era. Sinclair Oil featured advertisements in one hundred and four newspapers and five national magazines displaying a dozen different dinosaurs, from the menacing tyrannosaurus red and three-horned triceratops to the peace loving passive yet massive forty ton vegetarian Apatosaurus (brontosaurus) with a tail thirty feet long. Sinclair used 'Dino' a big green Apatosaurus (Brontosaurus) as its official mascot and corporate symbol, trademarking the dinosaur in 1932.

P. G. Allen, developer of life-like papier-mâché animals for the motion picture industry, was working on an exhibit for the 1933 Century of Progress Exposition in Chicago, the equivalent of a World Fair. Sinclair Oil sponsored the dinosaur exhibition and to enhance the academic stature of its promotions financed the dinosaur-fossil search expeditions of Dr. Barnum Brown, curator at the American Museum of Natural History. After Doctor Brown's death in January 1963, Sinclair retained Dr. John H. Ostrom of Yale University's Peabody Museum of Natural History as consultant on the Sinclair sponsored Paleontology exhibit at New York World's Fair in 1964.

Sinclair's marketing was a masterstroke, but led to the common public misperception that petroleum is predominantly derived from the organic remains of the great dinosaurs. Rather than the enormous dinosaurs, it was microscopic bacteria that produced the petroleum reserves if our time period. Single-celled bacteria evolved in the earth's oceans about three billion years ago, and were the dominant life form on the planet until about 600 million years ago. In fact, if dominant is qualified as largest by biomass, bacteria retain that distinction today.

As microscopic as the individual bacteria may be, the bacterial colonies known as "mats" were of enormous proportions. They had masses of millions of tons compared to the hundred tons for the largest dinosaur, the sauropods. As these massive colonies died off and decayed they subsided to the bottom of the sea and were covered by layers of accumulating sediments. Over millions of years these layers of sediment thousands of feet underground were compressed under tremendous pressure and temperature, and developed into the liquid hydrocarbons we recognize as petroleum.

The vast majority of the world's coal deposits date back to the Carboniferous period, about three hundred million years ago. The first dinosaurs would not make their grand entrance in the evolutionary timetable until seventy-five million years later. During the Carboniferous period the earth was heavily forested. With the death and decomposition of these trees and plant life buried under great pressure and temperature under heavy layers of sediment, they were transformed into solid coal rather than liquid petroleum. As the search for petroleum and coal preserves often entails drilling and excavation of deep layers of sediment, it is not uncommon for fossils of dinosaurs and other prehistoric forms of life to be uncovered. The discovery of a theropod dinosaur during fossil fuel exploration in China has been given the appropriate name Gasosaurus. It looks as though Dino's story may have come full circle.

Microbiology

The microbes of the gastrointestinal flora are major contributors to intestinal gas. Although unseen, an invisible world had been theorized for centuries. The ancient Greeks thought about it and wrote comprehensively about a world of atoms, molecules, and microscopic life forms far beyond the technology of their day. The glass lens makers from the thirteenth through sixteenth centuries provably developed ever improving prototypes of the microscope after first developing the telescope. It was only in the late 1674 that Antoine Van Leeuwenhoek, a glass lens maker, used an improved optical microscope of his own design to identify red blood cells, spermatozoa, and microorganisms. His advance began the field of microbiology, brining a previously invisible world into view. The field continues to bring new discoveries and understanding of life on earth and the interdependence of various life forms.

Microorganisms gave been found to survive and thrive in extreme locations from many miles underground in rocks, under the ice of Antarctica, in volcanic vents under seas, and the vacuum of outer space. The world of microorganisms has expanded from knowledge of bacteria, to discovery of other microorganisms such as the virus, prion, and Archaea. The future will probably yield further discoveries as continuing research and advancing technology allow.

From the time of Van Leeuwenhoek to the present dramatic advances have taken place in the understanding of the role of microorganisms in human health and disease, as well as life in general. Louis Pasteur was a pioneering influence and identified the role of microorganisms in the fermentation process leading to enhanced production of wine, cheese, and vinegar. He developed an immunization program to protect cattle from anthrax, as well as to treat people exposed to the previously uniformly fatal rabies. He was able to disprove the prevailing theory of spontaneous generation of life and developed the process of disabling most pathogenic organisms by boiling in a process that was named after him, pasteurization.

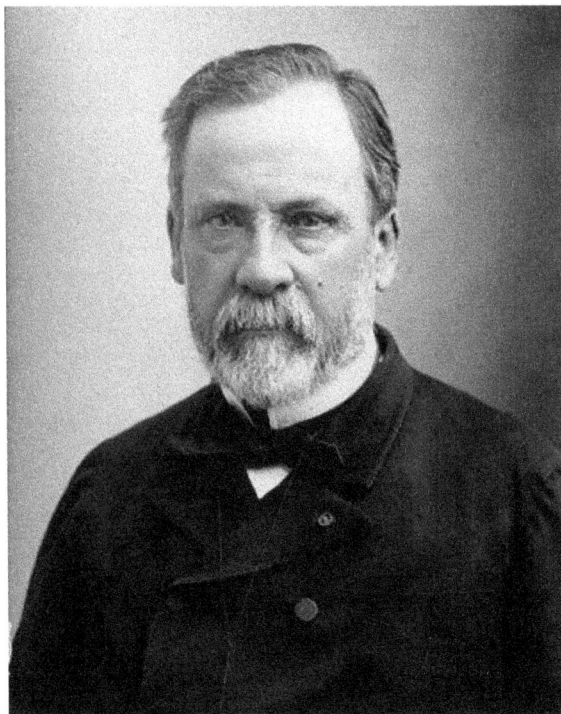

Louis Pasteur, Public Domain

It took many more years for the concept of pathogenic organisms to bring hygiene to a new level of awareness. Even in medical circles there was great reluctance to embrace hand washing and the use of disinfectants. Joseph Lister was preceded by Ignatz Semmelweis who fought an ignorant medical establishment that used to operate on trusting patients with their bare hands. Semmelweis was able to prove that infections were transmitted from the autopsy room to the operating room because hands were not washed. In spite of this proof he was ignored and ridiculed, which led to his mental collapse and death in a psychiatric hospital because he could not save thousands of innocent people who were condemned to death because of arrogance and ignorance.

Similar stories can be found in many areas of science and medicine where lifesaving advances were delayed for decades or centuries. The story of anesthesia is a prime example where excruciatingly painful and gruesome surgeries were performed on awake subjects who were forcibly restrained, while the anesthetic of nitrous oxide was being used as laughing gas purely for entertainment purposes. The discoverer of nitrous oxide, Sir Humphrey Davies, an esteemed scientist suggested that it be studied as an anesthetic but the physicians and surgeons of his day simply ignored him. The rediscovery of it and other products as anesthetics is a remarkable story that has been told by several books on the subject.

Another interesting aspect of the story of microbiology is how it took hundreds of years for scientists and physicians to recognize that pathogenic organisms were responsible for many diseases. It has also taken a similar period of time for the recognition that ,most organisms are not pathogenic but are commensals ort actually improve health. One of the pioneers in this investigation was a scientist working at the Pasteur Institute in Paris, Dr. Élie Metchnikoff (1845-1916). He investigated the extreme longevity of centenarians in Bulgaria and believed their long lives were due to the yogurt and sour milk consumed as a regular part of their diet.

He received the Nobel Prize in Medicine for his work on immunity, and identified the *Lactobacillus delbrueckii subspecies bulgaricus* organism in yogurt that is considered an ideal probiotic. His theory of aging being due to toxic bacteria, and that lactic acid producing organisms could prolong life, were very influential. His advocacy of probiotics was embraced by the Japanese scientist Minoru Shirota who developed a stronger strain of the probiotic organism *Lactobacillus casei* found in Yakult and kefir. Dr. John Harvey Kellogg, the medical director of the Battle Creek Sanitarium, also embraced Dr. Metchnikoff's theory. Dr. Kellogg administered series of colonics to cleanse the bowels then had his patients eat half a bowl of yogurt, with the other half administered as an enema. Dr. Kellogg also advocated a high fiber high roughage diet and developed a corn flake cereal, founding the very successful Kellogg Cereal Company

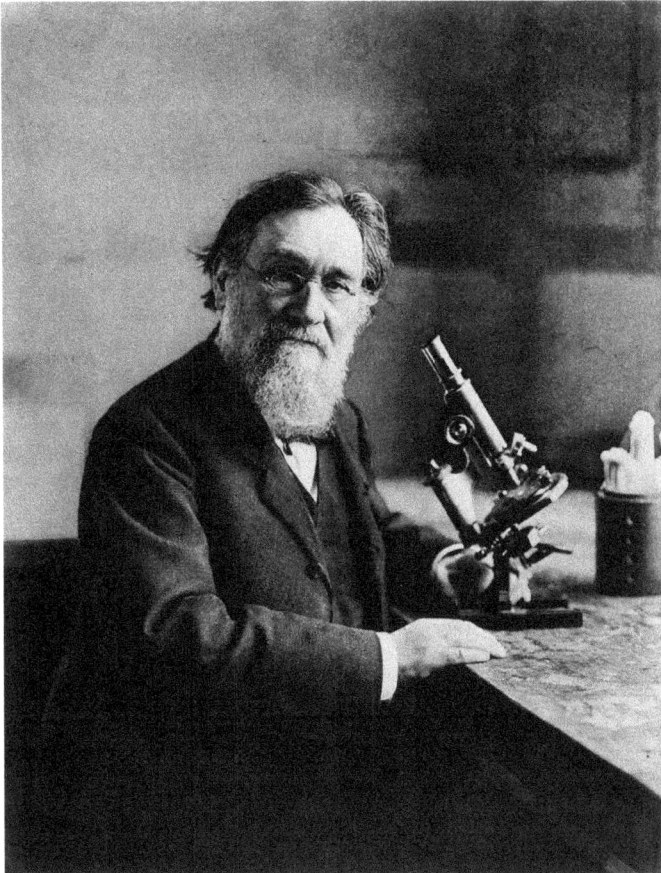

Élie Metchnikoff, Nobel Prize winning scientist at the Pasteur Institute in Paris

Unfortunately science and medicine are replete with many instances where personality flaws, greed, arrogance, jealousy, stupidity, ignorance, and a hundred and one other human failings led to missed opportunities to prevent or cure disease, and improve human health. Even more unfortunately these failings show no sign of abating, with conflicts of interest, desire for personal financial gain, overreaching for recognition, and the securing of patents, too often leading to fraud and deception. Of course dedicated and compassionate professionals are the majority, but progress is hindered nonetheless leading to the illness and death of innocents.

Microbiome

The micro biome includes microbes, their genomes, and their environmental interactions. Gut flora consists of the microorganisms that live in the digestive tract and are the largest component of the human flora. The gut flora contains approximately one hundred trillion microorganisms in its intestines, a number much greater than the ten trillion cells of the human body. The gut flora has approximately one hundred times as many genes as the human genome.

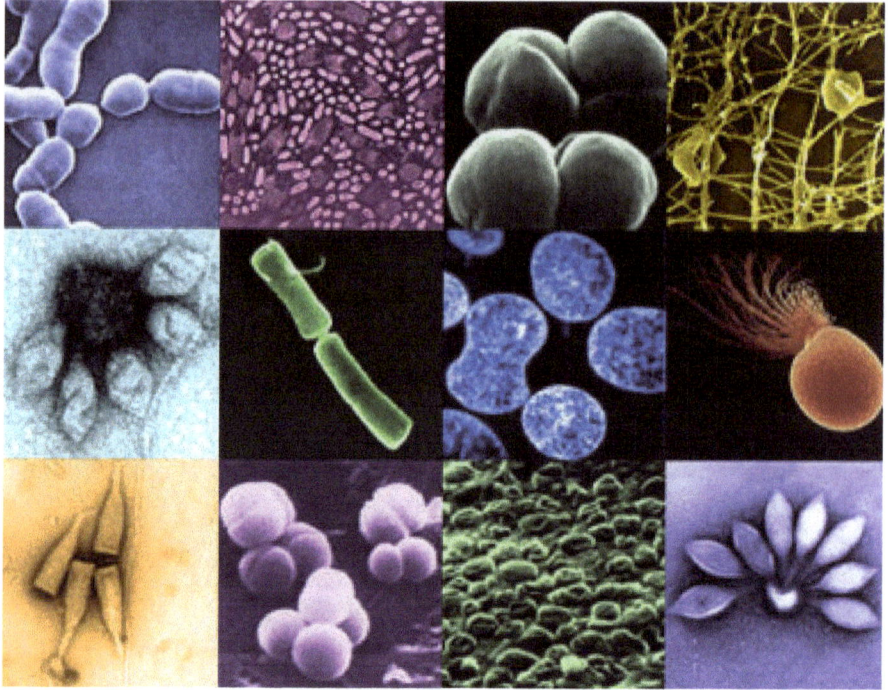

The human genome has twenty three thousand genomes and the human microbiome genome exceeds over one million and still counting. Any one or combination of these genomes, human and/or microbial, can play a very important role in health and disease. Alterations in an individual's flora may occur with changes in lifestyle, diet, illness, and age. The National Institutes of Health has embarked on the Human Microbiome Project to identify the organisms present in the human microbiome and their role in health and disease.

Anaerobic bacteria make up most of the flora in the colon and up to sixty percent of the dry mass of feces. These bacteria perform a variety of metabolic activities that benefit the host, so much so that some scientists refer to it as the "forgotten" organ. Their metabolic activity includes extracting energy from undigested carbohydrates by fermentation and absorption of short chain fatty acids. They also synthesize vitamin B and vitamin K as well as metabolizing bile acids and lipids. The gut flora also prevents pathogens from colonizing the intestines through competitive exclusion, also known as the "barrier effect". The bacteria stimulate the immune system lymphoid tissue to produce antibodies to pathogens, and to recognize and not develop an immune response to beneficial flora.

The human microbiome is normally established only after birth. Fetuses do accumulate a mass of sterile and odorless greenish feces called meconium, in their intestines. Fetuses usually pass meconium after birth but approximately twelve percent of pregnancies have yellow or green bile pigmented meconium stained amniotic fluid. The risk increases with the length of the pregnancy. In births occurring after forty-two weeks, described as post term, the rate of meconium staining approaches fifty percent. Fetuses have amniotic fluid in their lungs until they take their first breath of air after birth. In a minority of meconium stained amniotic fluid cases potentially fatal meconium aspiration syndrome occurs. If the newborn fails to pass meconium, a congenital abnormality of the colon needs to be excluded. Hirschsprung disease may involve failure of fetal development of the ganglions of the enteric nervous system. When it involves the colon, the bowel may not relax to allow the passage of meconium or feces and surgery may be required to remove the affected segment of bowel.

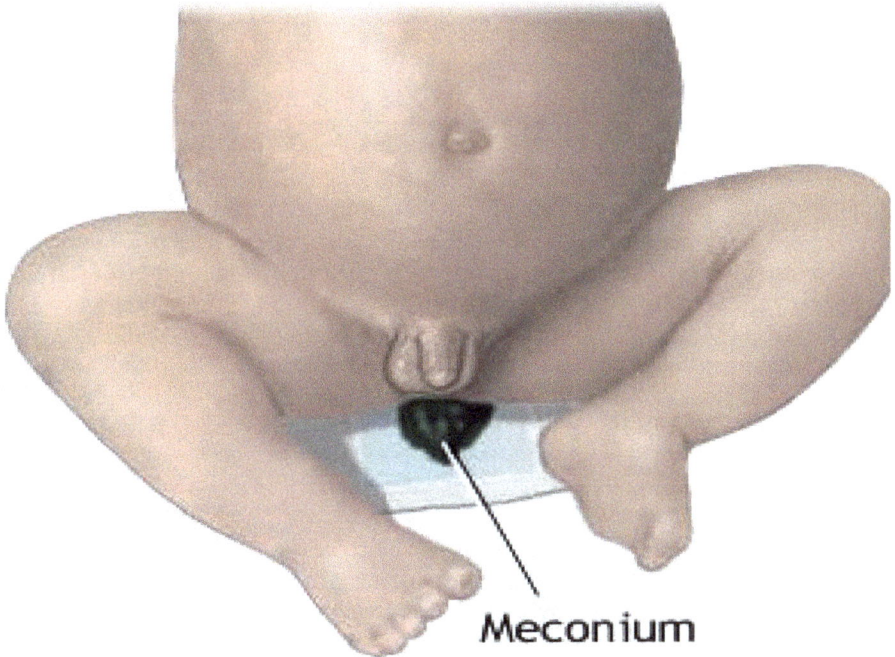

Meconium

www.healthcentral.com Creative Commons License

Since the digestive tract of the newborn is sterile, there are no microorganisms generating gas through cellular metabolism. All of the gas the newborn infant begins to pass is swallowed air. If an infant is bottle-fed rather than breast-fed they are much more likely to swallow even more air. Baby bottles are a common cause of aerophagia in infants as they suck in and swallow air if the formula does not always cover the nipple. Burping the baby after a feeding is the means of allowing the swallowed air to escape otherwise it will cause distension and discomfort. Some bottles are designed to use an internal plastic sleeve to prevent air from reaching the nipple when the formula is depleted the sleeve forms a vacuum so the infant is not sucking in air.

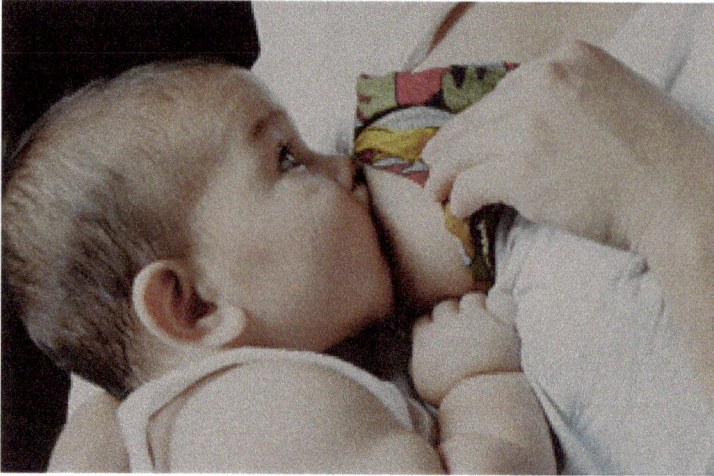

The first exposure to microorganism that will be swallowed and begin to colonize the infant digestive tract are from the birth mother if the delivery is vaginal and breast-feeding is initiated. The microorganisms that colonize the infant become its microbiome and play a major role in its ongoing health and wellness. The initial gut flora of the infant if born via a vaginal delivery and breast-feeding is identical to the vaginal and skin microbiome of the mother. This initial flora changes over the next few months especially if formula and other milks and foods are introduced. At about three months of age the gut flora is well established, and although changes will occur it is similar to the gut flora it will have as an adult.

The gut flora helps to set the infant's immune system, and it recognizes and tolerates microorganisms that are beneficial known as commensals. One of the theories why breast-feeding is preferable, as well as why a vaginal delivery is preferable to Caesarian section, is the natural microbiome exposure has advantages. The immunity of infants who did receive the natural microbiome from the mother is at a disadvantage. Some experts are advocating exposing the newborn to the mother's vaginal secretions and microbiome if the birth is via a Caesarian section.

The gut flora is one aspect of the microbiome, with skin, ears, mouth, genitourinary, and every surface of the body exposed to the external environment developing its own unique microbiome. Infants born by Caesarean section have exposure to different organisms, which establish a microbiome that is not believed to be as beneficial as via a natural vaginal delivery.

The microbiome is established rapidly upon exposure to the environment. Most people think that the digestive tract is an internal organ because it is located inside the body. They are often surprised to find out that that the digestive tract is actually considered an organ exposed to the external environment. It is a long hollow tube exposed to the external environment at both ends, and is transited by material that for the most part comes from outside of the body.

The results of cell division and multiplication are similar between cells of the body, and cells of the microbiome. Mathematically this growth pattern is described as exponential or logarithmic growth. For those more familiar with finance, it is more akin to compounding interest instead of simple arithmetic addition. If a single cell divides into two cells, those cells divide into four cells, those into eight cells, and the numbers increase rapidly. The colonization and establishment of the microbiome is extremely rapid. The limitation of cellular division and growth of human cells are controlled by genes, hormones, neurotransmitters, and a variety of other feedback control mechanisms. The microbiome is also under the influence of these mechanisms, as well as competition for habitat and nutrition.

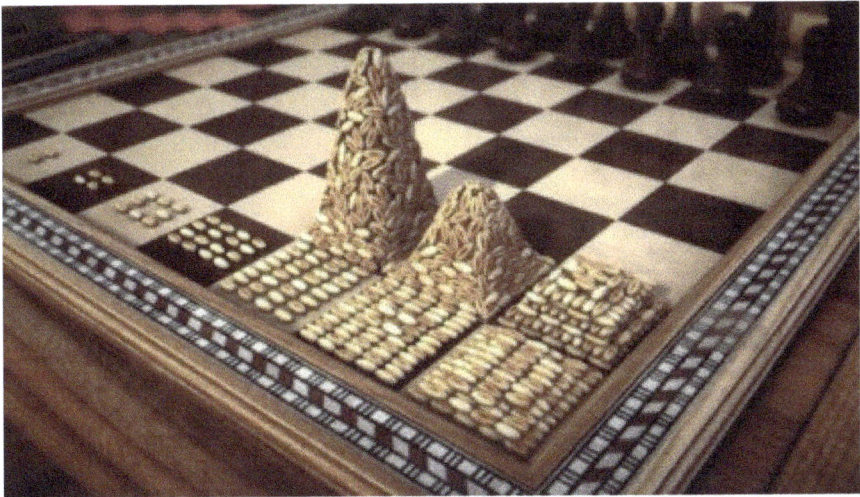

There is an apocryphal tale told of the invention of the game of chess. Long ago in an ancient land, there lived a very wise man that happened to be the Vizier at the court of a great Sultan. Months and years passed by and the great Sultan died, and his young prince replaced him. Being young, the prince lacked experience. He started spending more than what his father used to. The wise Vizier decided to teach the brash prince a lesson! The prince set a contest and as a reward, decided to give the winner whatever he wishes, boasting of his wealth, being under the illusion that his wealth is virtually endless. The Vizier won, and asked the prince for the prize: a single grain of wheat and a chessboard!

"What?! Just a grain of wheat! Are you insulting my wealth?" yelled the prince. "No! Your majesty!" The Vizier explained. "You have to promise to double that grain of wheat until the chessboard is full, so on the first day you give me one grain of wheat on the first square of the chessboard, on the second day you double it on the second square (giving me two grains), on the third, you double that on the third square (giving me four grains), and so on, until the sixty fourth square on the chessboard." "I would thought you being so smart", the young prince said. "You would ask for something more substantial. Anyway, if this is your wish I will grant you that."

And so, on the second day, the Vizier got 2 grains, on the third, he got 4 grains, and the young prince couldn't help himself making fun of the Vizier.
By the sixth day, the Vizier got 32 grains of wheat. By the eighth day and the end of the first row, he got a mere 128 grains. By the sixteenth day and the end of the second row, he got 32,768 grains. By the end of the game the prince could not provide enough grains to give the Vizier a chessboard's worth of grains because of the power of exponential growth. The last (sixty-fourth) square alone required 9,223,372,036,854,775,808 grains. The cumulative total of all of the squares was 18,446,744,073,709,551,615 grains. Indeed, that many grains would cover the entire earth several inches deep!

The gastrointestinal microbiome is also known as the gut microbiome and the gut flora. The gut microbiome is much more important than most people give it credit for. The microbes of the body far outnumber the number of human cells. The vast majorities are commensals or are engaged with us in a symbiotic relationship from which we both benefit. The normal flora is site specific so that the microbiome of the stomach is different from the small intestine, which is different again from the colon. The appendix serves as a reservoir of the normal large intestinal bacteria flora. It represents the healthy gut microbiome from which the gut flora can be replenished after a bout of intestinal dysentery.

The effect of the microbiome includes microbes, their genomes, and their environmental interactions. Gut flora consists of the microorganisms that live in the digestive tract and are the largest component of the human flora. The gut flora contains approximately one-hundred-trillion microorganisms in the intestinal tract, a number much greater than the ten trillion cells of the human body. The gut flora has approximately one hundred times as many genes as the human genome.

The human genome has twenty-three thousand genes and the human microbiome genome exceeds over one million genes and still counting. Any one or combination of these genes, human and/or microbial, can play a very important role in health and disease. Alterations in an individual's flora may occur with changes in lifestyle, diet, illness, and age. The National Institutes of Health has embarked on the Human Microbiome Project to identify the organisms present in the human microbiome and their role in health and disease.

Anaerobic bacteria make up most of the microbial flora of the colon and up to sixty percent of the dry mass of feces. These microorganisms perform a variety of metabolic activities that benefit the host, so much so that some scientists refer to it as the 'forgotten organ'. Their metabolic activity includes extracting energy from undigested carbohydrates by fermentation and absorption of short chain fatty acids. They also synthesize vitamin B and vitamin K, as well as metabolizing bile acids and lipids.

The gut flora also prevents pathogens from colonizing the intestines through competitive exclusion, also known as the 'barrier effect'. The bacteria stimulate the immune system lymphoid tissue to produce antibodies to pathogens, and to recognize and not develop an immune response to beneficial flora. One of the major advances in the understanding of microbial life has come about with the recent advances in genomics technology. This technology now allows the rapid and precise identification of organisms that could not be identified because they were too fastidious and difficult to culture from stool specimens.

These advances include the discovery of extremophiles, organisms that can live in extreme environments, and represent a previously undiscovered form of life called Archaea. This has prompted a reevaluation of the biological system of taxonomy, the categorizing of life forms. Most scientists now recognize six separate kingdoms: Animals (Animalia), Plants (Plantae), Fungi, Bacteria, Protozoan (Protista), and Archaea.

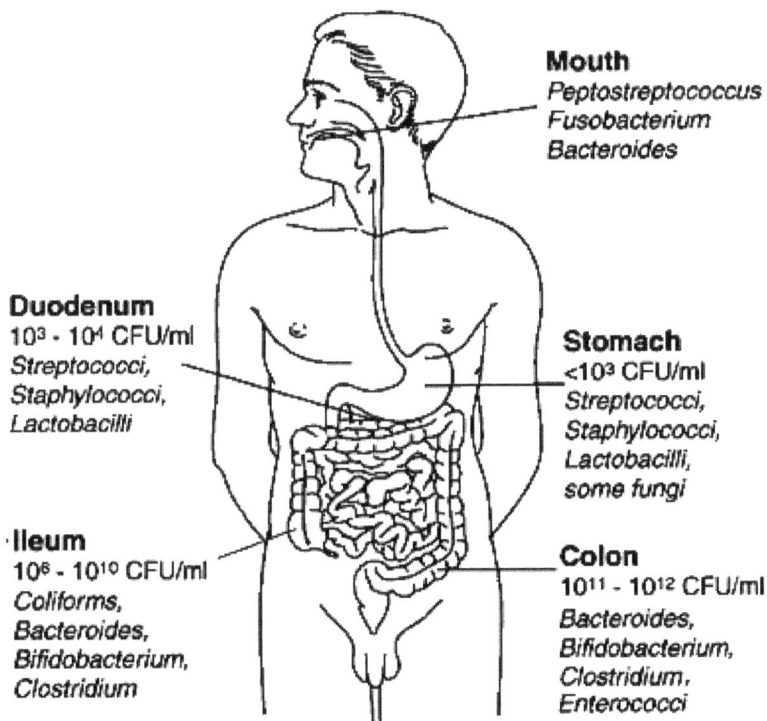

Mouth
Peptostreptococcus
Fusobacterium
Bacteroides

Duodenum
10^3 - 10^4 CFU/ml
Streptococci,
Staphylococci,
Lactobacilli

Stomach
$<10^3$ CFU/ml
Streptococci,
Staphylococci,
Lactobacilli,
some fungi

Ileum
10^6 - 10^{10} CFU/ml
Coliforms,
Bacteroides,
Bifidobacterium,
Clostridium

Colon
10^{11} - 10^{12} CFU/ml
Bacteroides,
Bifidobacterium,
Clostridium,
Enterococci

trialx.com/curetalk/wp Creative Commons License

Significant portions of the human microbiome are not bacteria at all and are actually Archaea. In fact, the methane produced in flatus comes from the methanogenic Archaea of the colon's microbiome. There will undoubtedly be major advances in the understanding of human health and diseases as the microbiome is explored and understood. The hygiene hypothesis proposes that a lack of early childhood exposure to infectious agents, parasites, and symbiotic microorganisms in the gut flora suppresses the development of the immune system. It is proposed that allergies, autoimmune disorders, and diseases seen at higher rates in the developed world may be due to excessive hygiene preventing the exposure necessary for optimal health. The hygiene hypothesis is supported by epidemiological data, yet the topic remains controversial with extensive research ongoing.

As a result of the hygiene hypothesis, helminthic infections emerged as a possible explanation of the low incidence of immunological disorders and autoimmune diseases in less developed countries. Helminthic therapy is the treatment of autoimmune diseases and immune disorders by means of deliberate infestation with a roundworm parasite. It is currently being studied as a promising treatment for several (non-viral) autoimmune diseases including Crohn disease, multiple sclerosis, asthma, and ulcerative colitis. The anti-inflammatory effects of helminth infection are also prompting research into diseases that are not currently considered to have an immune basis. For example, heart disease and arteriosclerosis both have similar epidemiological and inflammatory profiles to the autoimmune diseases. Presently the two versions of helminthic therapy being studied are *Trichuris suis* ova and *Necator americanus* larvae.

Dysbiosis (dysbacteriosis) refers to a condition with microbial imbalances on or inside the body. Dysbiosis is most prominent in the digestive tract or on the skin, but can also occur on any surface or mucous membrane exposed to the environment such as the vagina, lungs, mouth, nose, sinuses, ears, nails, or eyes. It has been associated with different illnesses, such as inflammatory bowel disease, as imbalances in the intestinal microbiome may be associated with bowel inflammation and chronic fatigue syndrome. Microbial colonies found on or in the body are normally benign or beneficial. These beneficial and appropriately sized microbial colonies carry out a series of helpful and necessary functions, such as aiding in digestion. They also protect the body from the penetration of and infection with pathogenic microbes. These beneficial microbial colonies compete with each other for space and resources.

When this balance is disturbed by any of a variety of causes, such as antibiotic exposure, the balance of the microbial populations becomes disturbed. This can lead to an overgrowth of one or more of the organisms, which then may have a negative effect on some of the beneficial organisms. The imbalance and negative impacts can initiate a vicious cycle with further disruption from the normal flora.

Small intestinal bacterial overgrowth (SIBO) is a disorder of excessive bacterial growth in the small bowel. Risk factors included decreased motility or anatomical changes that lead to stasis, immune deficiencies, and reflux of bacteria from the colon into the small bowel such as the surgical removal of the ileocecal valve. The symptoms of bacterial overgrowth may include nausea, vomiting, bloating, flatus, chronic diarrhea, constipation, abdominal discomfort, weight loss, malnutrition, and anemia from vitamin B_{12} deficiency. Irritable bowel syndrome (IBS) may have an association with small intestinal bacterial overgrowth with some studies showing improvement after treatment. Rosacea, a dermatological condition, also appears to have an association with improvement after treatment. Small bowel bacterial overgrowth syndrome is treated with antibiotics, and if retreatment is required, various antibiotics may be given in a cyclic fashion.

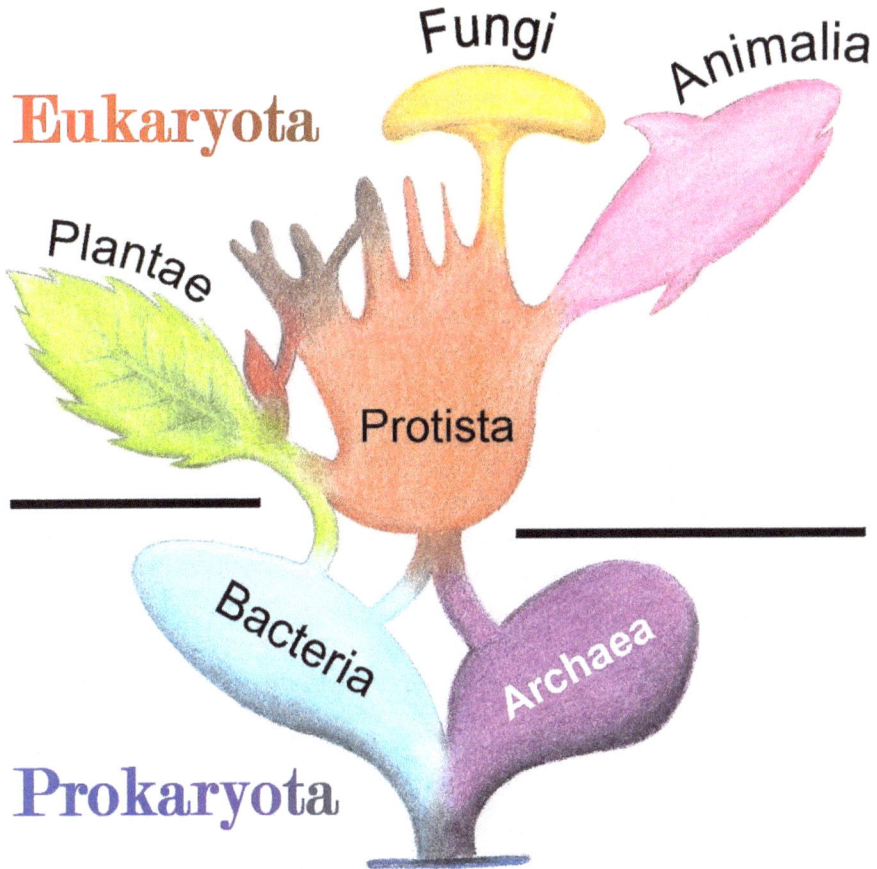

Maulucioni y Dorid Creative Commons License

Archaea

Phylogenetics was proposed in 1965 by Linus Pauling and Emile Zuckerlan using the sequences of the genes in organisms to determine how they are related to each other. Archaea were first classified as a separate group of prokaryotes in 1977 by Carl Woese and George E. Fox in phylogenetic trees based on the sequences of ribosomal ribonucleic acid (rRNA) genes. Archaea were first found in extreme environments, such as volcanic hot springs. The word *archaea* comes from the Ancient Greek ἀρχαῖα, meaning 'ancient things' as the first representatives of the domain Archaea were methanogens and it was assumed that their metabolism reflected Earth's primitive atmosphere and the organism's antiquity. Archaea (singular *archaeon*) are prokaryote microorganisms, meaning that they have no cell nucleus or any other membrane-bound organelles in their cells. Archaeal cells have unique properties separating them from the other two domains of life: Bacteria and Eukaryota.

Archaea and bacteria are generally similar in size and shape, although a few Archaea have very strange shapes, such as flat and square-shaped cells. Despite a visual similarity to bacteria, Archaea possess genes and several metabolic pathways that are more closely related to those of eukaryotes. Archaea use more energy sources than eukaryotes. These range from organic compounds, such as sugars, ammonia, metal ions, hydrogen sulfide, elemental sulfur, and hydrogen gas. They can also utilize light without photosynthesis in a process known as photophosphorylation in salt-tolerant Archaea. Archaea reproduce asexually by binary fission, fragmentation, or budding.

Archaea were initially viewed as extremophiles living in extremely harsh environments, such as hot mineral springs, volcanic vents, salt lakes, and in glaciers. They have since been found in a broad range of habitats, including non-extreme environments such as soils, oceans, marshes, and the human colon and navel. Archaea are particularly plentiful in the oceans and in plankton. Archaea may play major roles in both the carbon and nitrogen cycles. There are no known examples of Archaea acting as pathogens or parasites. Archaea can also be commensals, benefiting from an association without helping or harming the other organism.

They are often found in the role of mutualism with a symbiotic benefit for both organisms. One example of mutualism are the methanogens found in the digestive tracts where they aid digestion. In anaerobic environments within ruminants and termites, cellulose is broken down by protozoans with the release of hydrogen gas. The Archaea methanogens reside within the protozoan and convert the hydrogen to methane within the protozoans organelle known as a hydrogenosome. Methanogens are also used in biogas production and sewage treatment. The heat stable enzymes from extremophile Archaea are used in biotechnology.

Archaea also associate with larger organisms such as corals, plant roots, and even in humans. For example, the methanogen *Methanobrevibacter smithii* comprises ten percent of the prokaryotes in the human gut flora. Archaea demonstrate a high level of horizontal gene transfer between species. The mitochondria which serve as the energy power source for human cells is thought to have originated as an independent organism that entered into a symbiotic relationship

Archaea are a relatively recent discovery that has revolutionized our understanding of the microbial world and in particular the human microbiome. One of the major advances in the understanding of microbial life has come about with the recent advances in genomics technology. This has been the discovery of extremophiles, organisms that can live in extreme environments and represented a previously undiscovered form of life called Archaea. This has prompted a reevaluation of the biological system of taxonomy, the categorizing of life forms. Most scientists now recognize six separate kingdoms: Animals (Animalia), Plants (Plantae), Fungi, Bacteria, Protozoan (Protista), and Archaea.

Significant portions of the human micro biome are not bacteria at all and are actually Achaea. In fact the methane produced in flatus comes from the methanogenic Achaea of the colon's microbiome. Intense research activities are now being undertaken by the National Institute of health to identify and categorize the species and understand the activities of the flora in the Human Microbiome Project. There will undoubtedly be major advances in the understanding of human health and diseases as the micro biome is explored and understood.

Most people have not heard of the microorganisms called Archaea, which is a kingdom of single-celled microorganisms that have no cell nucleus or membrane-bound organelles within their cells. They were first discovered in extremely hot and acidic environments in which life was not thought possible to exist. It was like a science fiction story come to life that not only were organisms found to survive in this environment but also they were actually thriving in these extreme conditions. In the late 1970's, Dr. Carl Woese at the University of Illinois at Urbana Champaign used RNA sequences to determine how closely these newly discovered microbes were to other bacteria. He discovered that the prokaryotes were actually composed of two entirely different groups, the bacteria and a newly recognized group that he called Archaea. These three groups are now recognized as the three distinct domains of life.

Archaea and bacteria have a similar size and shape, which may have delayed their recognition as completely separate entities. Although a few Achaea have strange and unusual shapes, most look indistinguishable from bacteria by visual appearance. Their genetics and biochemistry are unique and there is no question but that they are an entirely different form of life. Archaea reproduce asexually by binary fission, fragmentation, or budding; unlike bacteria and eukaryotes, no known species form spores.

Initially, Achaea were thought to be limited to extremophiles having been found in geysers, deep ocean black smokers, and oil wells. Other extreme habitats included very cold art tic waters, and highly saline, acidic, or alkaline water. They have since been found in a wide variety of habitats including of soils, oceans, marshes, and the human colon and navel. Archaea are abundant in the oceans and may be active in both the carbon and the nitrogen cycle. They may represent up to twenty percent of the earths entire biomass.

Even acids with the extreme limit of a pH of zero were tolerable environments. Temperatures higher than that of boiling water which was thought to sterilize and kill al bacteria was comfortable for their reproduction. In fact they would survive in an environment as hostile as the planet Mars. Some scientists postulate that the first Achaea may have arrived on Earth on a meteorite and are actually extraterrestrial life that cane to earth from another planet or outside of our solar system. Science fiction could not be any more exciting than the actual science of studying Archaea.

There are no Archaea pathogens or parasites known, and they are often they are often commensals. One example of commensalism is the methanogens that inhabit the digestive tracts of humans and ruminants where they aid digestion. Methanogens are the primary source of the methane in the atmosphere and are major contributors to global warming. They are also used in biogas production and sewage treatment. The enzymes from extremophile Achaea can endure high temperatures and organic solvents and have contributed to major advances in biotechnology, environmental services, and the food service industry.

Extremophile Archaea are a source of enzymes that function under harsh conditions if temperature, salinity, acidity, or alkalinity. These enzymes have found many uses including research and industry. As an example amylases and galactosidases that function at over 100 °C (212 °F) may allow food processing at higher temperatures that usual. This may have commercial applications in the production of low lactose milk and whey. Archaea may also be hosts to new classes of antibiotics.

Extremophiles & Psychrophiles (Cryophiles)

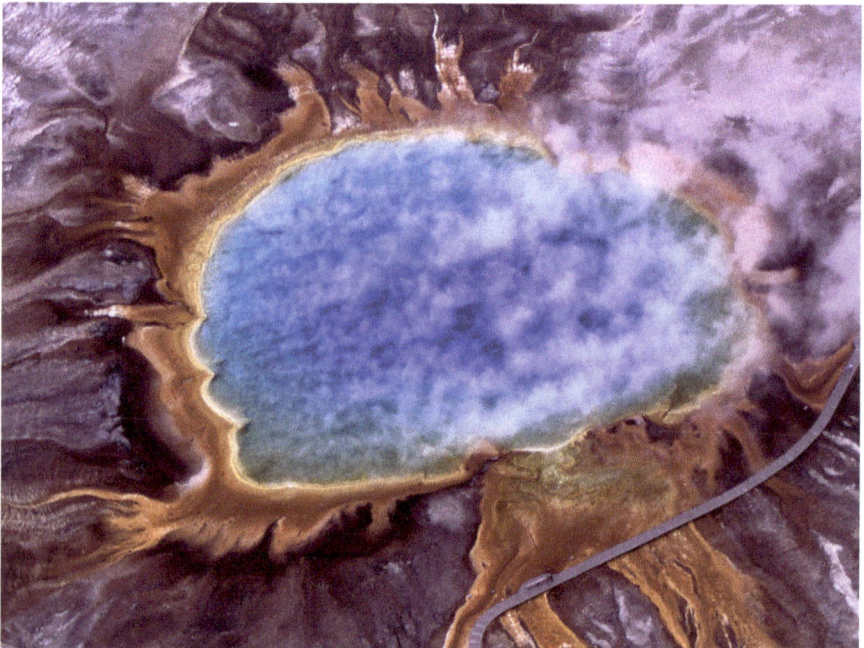

Grand Prismatic Mineral Hot Springs Yellowstone National Park. The striking coloration are from the extremophile Archaea that thrive in extreme environments that were previously thought to be incompatible with life. Creative Commons License

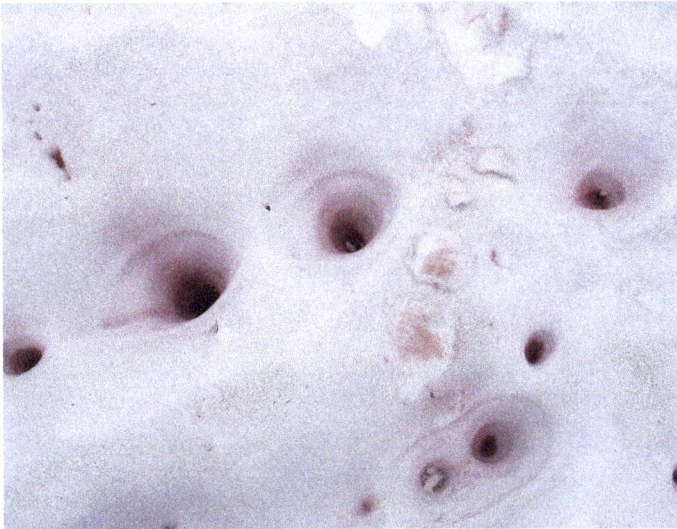

Unusual watermelon snow pits. 2206 Author Will Beback Creative Commons License

Psychrophiles also called cryophiles are extremophile organisms that are can successfully grow and reproduction in the cold temperature range from −15°C to +10°C. Temperatures as low as −15°C may be found in regions of high salinity water, known as brine, that is surrounded by sea ice. Thermophiles by contrast thrive at unusually hot temperatures. Psychrophiles are very adaptive and use a wide variety of metabolic pathways to survive. These include the processes of photosynthesis, chemoautotrophy (also known as lithotrophy), and heterotrophy. This adaptive strategy allows them to survive and thrive in diverse communities throughout the colder climate zones. They are found in diverse extreme environments including soil in alpine and arctic environments, deep ocean waters at very high latitudes, polar ice fields, glaciers, and snowfields.

They are of particular interest to astrobiology, the science of potential extraterrestrial life, and to geomicrobiology, the scientific study of microbes active in geochemical processes. In a research study at the University of Alaska Fairbanks a one thousand liter biogas digester using psychrophiles produces two hundred to three hundred liters of methane per day. Although it is only about twenty to thirty percent of the output from those in warmer climates, it is still a significant amount of biological activity in extreme cold climate zones. Most psychrophiles are either bacteria or Achaea present in widely diverse microbial lineages. Novel groups of psychrophilic fungi live in oxygen poor areas under alpine snowfields. Aristotle 384 BCE – 322 BCE wrote the first descriptive accounts of watermelon snow. It has puzzled mountain climbers, explorers, and naturalists for thousands of years.

The dramatic appearance of Watermelon snow, also called snow algae, red snow, or blood snow, is *Chlamydomonas nivalis* (Latin nivalis – snow), is the visible mark of the psychrophilic species of green algae. Compressing the snow by walking on it, or making snowballs, gives it a red color from a secondary red carotenoid pigment (astaxanthin), which it has in addition to chlorophyll. Psychrophiles have lipid cell membranes chemically resistant to the stiffening effect of extreme cold. They often create protein 'antifreezes' to maintain their intracellular space as liquid to protect their nuclear DNA in temperatures below the normal freezing point of water.

Methanogens

Methanogens are microorganisms of the Kingdom Archaea, not bacteria as previously thought. They produce methane as a metabolic byproduct in anaerobic conditions when oxygen is not present. Methanogens have been identified in a wide variety of extreme environments. Methanogens can thrive and reproduce in boiling water, as well as in ice cores taken miles down in arctic glaciers. They are common in wetlands, where they produce marsh gas, and in the digestive tracts of animals and humans where they generate the methane content of flatulence as well as the ruminant belch.

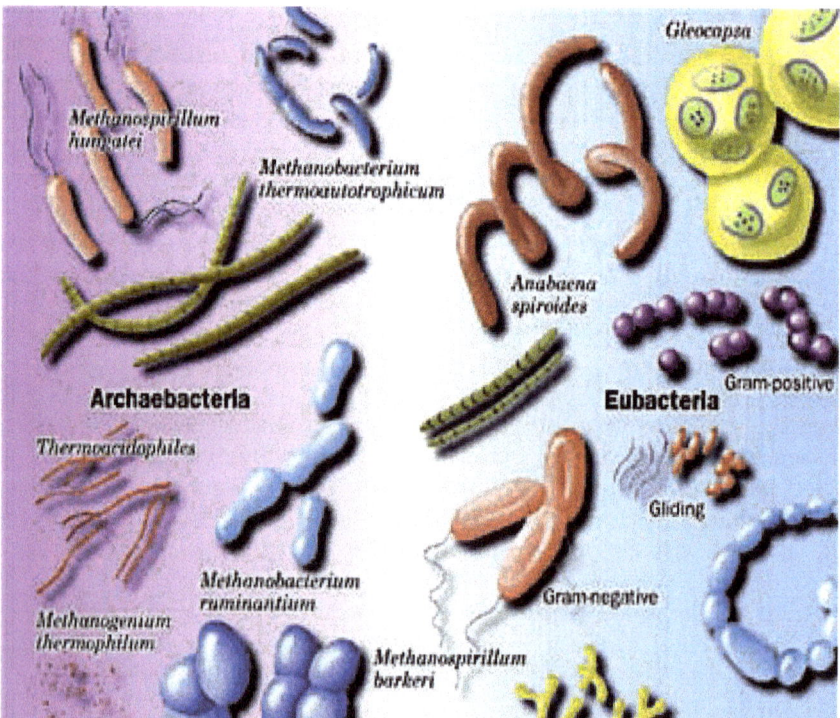

Most of the methanogenic bacteria are Archaea lawrencekok.blogspot.com Creative Commons License

Archaea are a relatively recent discovery that has revolutionized our understanding of the microbial world and in particular the human microbiome. One of the major advances in the understanding of microbial life has come about with the recent advances in genomics technology. This has been the discovery of extremophiles, organisms that can live in extreme environments and represented a previously undiscovered form of life called Archaea. This has prompted a reevaluation of the biological system of taxonomy, the categorizing of life forms. Most scientists now recognize six separate kingdoms: Animals (Animalia), Plants (Plantae), Fungi, Bacteria, Protozoan (Protista), and Archaea.

Significant portions of the human micro biome are not bacteria at all and are actually Achaea. In fact the methane produced in flatus comes from the methanogenic Achaea of the colon's micro biome. Intense research activities are now being undertaken by the National Institute of health to identify and categorize the species and understand the activities of the flora in the Human Microbiome Project. There will undoubtedly be major advances in the understanding of human health and diseases as the micro biome is explored and understood.

Most people have not heard of the microorganisms called Archaea, which is a kingdom of single-celled microorganisms that have no cell nucleus or membrane-bound organelles within their cells. They were first discovered in extremely hot and acidic environments in which life was not thought possible to exist. It was like a science fiction story come to life that not only were organisms found to survive in this environment but also they were actually thriving in these extreme conditions.

Bacteria

Bacteria (Greek bakterion rod) are categorized as a large kingdom of prokaryotic microorganisms. Typically just a few micrometers in length bacteria have a wide variety of shapes including, rods, spirals, and spheres. Bacteria were among the earliest forms of life to appear on Earth, and are ubiquitous. They inhabit soil, water, acidic hot springs, radioactive waste, and can reside deep within rocks miles underground in portions of Earth's crust. Bacteria also live inside of plants and animals and have survived in outer space during space flights. A gram of soil typically contains forty million bacterial cells and a single milliliter of fresh water may contain a million bacterial cells. There are approximately five nonillion, or to use a numerical version 5,000,000,000,000,000,000,000,000,000,000 (5×10 to the 30th power) bacteria on Earth. The enormous quantity of bacteria on Earth forms a total biomass that exceeds that of all plants and animals on the planet combined.

Bacteria are critical to life on Earth actively participating in many steps in the nutrient cycles that depend on these organisms, such as the fixation of nitrogen from the atmosphere. Most bacteria have yet to be identified and characterized. The science and study of bacteria is the field known as bacteriology, and is a branch of microbiology.

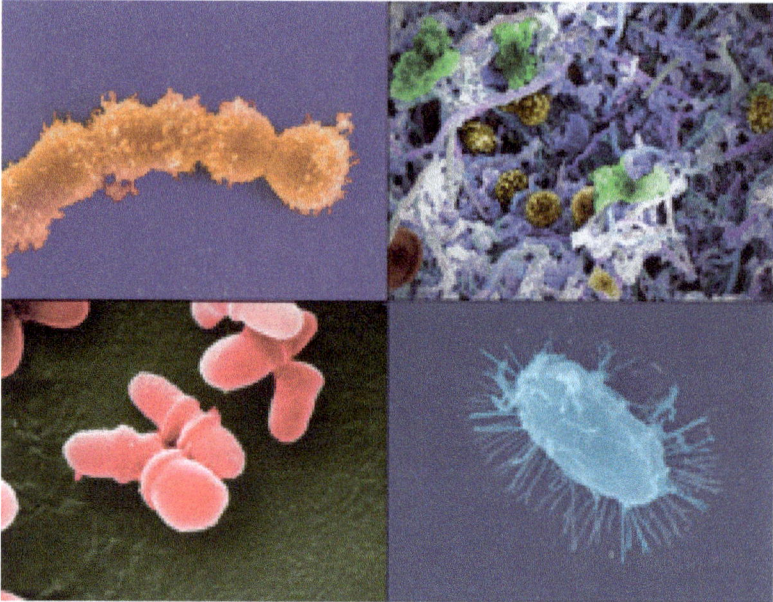

There are more than ten times as many bacterial cells in the human microbiome flora as there are human cells in the body. Very large numbers of bacteria are on the skin, and even more dramatic numbers are present as gut flora. The overwhelming majority of the bacteria in the body are commensals and do not cause disease. They are prevented from becoming pathogenic because of the protective effects of the immune system. Some bacteria are beneficial and engage in a symbiotic relationship with their human host.

Most people are not aware of the beneficial nature of the vast majority of bacteria. The recognition that several bacteria can be pathogenic and lead to disease and death has been well publicized. Several of the species of bacteria that are pathogenic and cause infectious diseases include cholera, syphilis, anthrax, leprosy, and bubonic plague. Many fatal bacterial diseases are respiratory infections, with tuberculosis alone killing about two million people a year. Antibiotics are utilized to treat bacterial infections, and are often also used in livestock farming. This has allowed antibiotic resistance to become increasingly common. In industry bacteria are important in sewage treatment, breakdown of oil spills, production of cheese and yogurt through fermentation. They have also been utilized in the mining industry in the recovery of gold, palladium, copper and other metals. Newer uses include biotechnology, the manufacture of antibiotics, and other proteins and chemicals.

Bacteria in the past were classified as plants in the class Schizomycetes. They are no longer considered members of the plant kingdom and at the present time bacteria are classified as prokaryotes. Prokaryotes are unlike the cells of animals and other eukaryotes. The cells of bacteria do not have a nucleus that contains the DNA based genetic information, and rarely have membrane bound organelles.

The term bacteria historically included all prokaryotes. About two decades ago a major scientific breakthrough occurred with the discovery that prokaryotes actually consist of two very different groups of organisms. They are presently classified as two distinct evolutionary kingdoms, Bacteria and Archaea. The prehistoric ancestors of both bacteria and Archaea were unicellular microorganisms that first appeared on Earth about four billion years ago. For about three billion years the dominant forms of life on Earth were microscopic bacteria and Archaea. Bacteria also played a major role in the evolutionary branching of eukaryotes from Archaea.

Eukaryotes developed from ancient bacteria physically entering the cells in an internally symbiotic association. This process, which began as the engulfment of symbiotic bacteria, progressed to the development of either mitochondria or hydrogenosomes. Some eukaryotes that already contained mitochondria that had previously developed from bacteria also engulfed cyanobacteria-like organisms. This symbiotic relationship developed into the formation of specialized chloroplasts in algae and plants.

Bacteria have a very wide diversity of shapes and sizes and are typically much smaller than eukaryotic cells. Most bacteria are between one half and five micrometers in length. The genus Mycoplasma has the smallest size of any bacteria, measuring only one third of a micrometer. They are so small that they are the same size as the largest viruses. Most bacterial species are either spherical cocci (Greek kókkos, grain) or rod shaped bacilli (Latin baculus stick). Elongation is commonly associated with motility. The bacteria called vibrio are rods with a slightly curved comma shape. Others bacteria called spirilla and spirochetes can be spiral shaped and tightly coiled. Several unusual species have a tetrahedral or cuboidal shape.

Recently discovered bacteria were identified deep under the Earth's crust. They grow as a branching filament with a star-shaped cross-section. These bacteria have a large surface area to volume ratio, which may be beneficial as these organisms exist in nutrient poor environments. A number of species of bacteria are found as single cells. Other species are often found in groups of multiple organisms that may associate in characteristic patterns. Neisseria organisms form pairs, Streptococcus organisms form chains, and Staphylococcus organisms group together in bunches and clusters that have the appearance of grapes. Less common species such as the genus Nocardia form complexes of branched filaments that have an appearance similar to that of fungal mycelia.

Bacteria frequently adhere to surfaces and may form a dense biofilm layer. These films may be as thin as just a few micrometers and may range up to thick bacterial mats up to half a meter in depth. These film layers and mats may contain a multitude of species of bacteria, protists, and Archaea. Many bacteria living in biofilms have a complex arrangement of both cells and extracellular components. These may form complex secondary structures comprising microcolonies with networks of channels to allow the diffusion of nutrients.

A lipid membrane known as a cell membrane or plasma membrane surrounds the bacterial cell. The cell membrane envelops and contains the contents of the cell. It acts as an environmental barrier and holds nutrients, proteins, and the other metabolically essential components of the cytoplasm within the cell. Bacteria, as prokaryotes, have few large intracellular structures and lack a true nucleus. They do not usually have membrane bound organelles in their cytoplasm such as mitochondria and chloroplasts that may be present in eukaryotic cells. Cyanobacteria may also produce gas within the cell, which forms into membrane bound vesicles. The gas vesicles may be used for locomotion by regulating their buoyancy. This allows the cell to move up or down in an aqueous environment, traveling to water layers with different light intensity and nutrient levels.

A special staining technique for the microscopic examination of bacteria was developed in 1884 by Hans Christian Gram. The Gram stain characterizes bacteria based on the structure of their cell walls. The thick layers of peptidoglycan and teichoic acids in the Gram-positive cell wall stain purple. The relatively thin Gram-negative cell wall consists of just a few layers of peptidoglycan. These layers are surrounded by a second lipid membrane containing lipoproteins and lipopolysaccharides appear pink. The endotoxin lipopolysaccharides are composed of lipid A and polysaccharides that contribute to the toxicity of Gram-negative bacteria.

A bacteria in which the cell wall has been entirely removed is called a protoplast. If the cell wall is partially removed it is called a spheroplast. ß-Lactam antibiotics, such as penicillin, interfere with the formation of peptidoglycan cross links disrupting the bacterial cell wall. The enzyme lysozyme, which is found in human tears, also disrupts and digests the cell wall of bacteria. This property of the tear lysozyme is the body's main defense against eye infections.

Swimming and motile bacteria frequently move between ten and one hundred body lengths per second. On a relative scale this makes them at least as fast as fish. Flagella are whip like rigid protein structures about twenty micrometers in length and twenty nanometers in diameter that are used for motility. Fimbriae are fine filaments of protein that are found all over the surface of the cell. They appear to be involved in the bacterial cell's ability to attach to solid surfaces or to other cells. The fimbriae are essential for the virulence of some pathogens. Pili are cellular appendages that are slightly larger than fimbriae and can transfer genetic material between bacterial cells in a process called conjugation in which they are called conjugation pili or sex pili.

Certain bacteria, such as Sporohalobacter, Clostridium, Heliobacterium, Anaerobacter, can form dormant structures that are highly resistant to destruction. These structures are called endospores and have a central cytoplasm core containing the DNA and ribosomes. They are surrounded by an impermeable and rigid protective coat. Endospores appear to be in a state of suspended animation and do not exhibit any signs of metabolic activity. They can survive extreme physical and chemical stresses that would kill metabolically active organisms. They have exhibited the ability to withstand high levels of UV light, gamma radiation, heat, freezing, detergents, disinfectants, pressure, desiccation, and outer space without any reduction in their pathogenicity. Endospores in this dormant state these organisms may remain viable for many millions of years. Viable spores that are over forty million years old have been identified that have maintained the ability to cause disease. Examples of disease caused by dormant spores include anthrax, which can be contracted by the inhalation of *Bacillus anthracis* endospores, and tetanus, which can be contracted by contamination of deep puncture wounds with *Clostridium tetani* endospores.

In unicellular organisms growth is manifested by increases in cell size until a fixed point where asexual reproduction by binary cell division takes place. Under ideal conditions bacteria can grow and undergo cell division very rapidly. Bacterial populations can double in size as quickly as every ten minutes. This exponential growth rate allows one cell to become 64 cells in one hour, 4,096 cells in two hours, 262,144 cells in three hours, 16,777,216 cells in four hours, over a billion cells in five hours, over four trillion cells in seven hours, etcetera. Certain infections can overwhelm and kill previously healthy humans and animals in a matter of just a few hours. The same power of exponential growth makes using microbes as miniature factories to produce biologic agents such as hormones, antibiotics, nutrients, etc. extremely attractive and efficient.

Bacteria are organisms that grow and multiply quickly. This feature, along with the relative ease to manipulate their DNA content, has made bacteria a model for many studies of genetics, molecular biology, and biochemistry. By creating a mutation in the DNA of bacteria a specific gene can be inactivated. By examining the effect of gene mutations, the function of genes, enzymes and metabolic pathways in bacteria can be identified. As many genes have identical functions in different organism the knowledge gained in experiments on bacteria can often be applied to more complex organisms such as humans. The scientific understanding of bacterial genes and metabolism has allowed the use of biotechnology to be commercialized. Bacteria can be bioengineered to produce a variety of therapeutic proteins, such as insulin, growth hormone, enzymes, antibodies, and other vital products.

Certain bacteria form close associations that are essential for their survival. One such mutualistic association occurs between anaerobic bacteria that metabolize a variety of organic acids. When organic acids such as butyric acid or propionic acid are metabolized hydrogen is produced as a byproduct. Increasing concentrations of hydrogen would be detrimental to the survival of these bacteria. In an association with mutual benefits methanogenic Archaea consume the hydrogen and allow the bacteria to thrive. The rhizosphere is the zone of soil that includes the root surface and soil that adheres to the root after gentle shaking. This zone contains a multitude of microorganisms that may carry out nitrogen fixation converting nitrogen gas to nitrogenous compounds. This provides an easily absorbable form of nitrogen for many plants, which cannot absorb and fix nitrogen from the atmosphere themselves.

There are many bacteria that have developed a symbiotic relationship with other organisms, including humans. In the human gastrointestinal tract, the gut flora also known as the microbiome, is predominantly beneficial organisms. There are over one thousand different species of bacteria in the normal human gut flora of the intestines. The organisms of the normal gut flora may contribute to gut immunity, synthesize vitamins such as vitamin K, folic acid, and biotin, convert sugars to lactic acid (Lactobacillus), as well as ferment complex indigestible carbohydrates. The presence of the normal gut flora inhibits potentially pathogenic bacteria from becoming established by the process of competitive exclusion. Supplements of beneficial bacteria may be provided as probiotic dietary supplements.

Pathogenic bacteria are the cause of a number of human diseases that may lead to illness and death and cause infections such as diphtheria, tetanus, syphilis, typhoid fever, leprosy, tuberculosis, cholera, and foodborne illness. A number of known medical diseases were discovered to be caused by pathogenic bacteria many decades or centuries after the disease was first described. A recent example was the discovery that peptic ulcer disease, long thought to be caused by excess gastric acidity, was actually caused by the pathogenic organism *Helicobacter pylori*. Bacterial diseases are also have a major impact on agriculture with bacteria causing fire blight, leaf spot, and wilts in plants, as well as mastitis, anthrax, Johne disease, and salmonella and in farm animals.

A number of species may exist in small numbers within the normal gut flora and microbiome. They become pathogenic and cause disease with a characteristic pattern of signs and symptoms when their numbers increase substantially. Some organisms can cause a variety of signs and symptoms dependent on the location of the infection. For example, Staphylococcus or Streptococcus can cause skin infections, pneumonia, meningitis and even overwhelming sepsis. Sepsis is a systemic inflammatory response that can lead to vascular collapse and death. At the same time, in smaller numbers, these organisms are part of the normal human microbiome that is present on the skin or in the nose without causing any illness.

Microorganisms have been utilized by humans for thousands of years in food production and preparation. Lactic acid is a metabolic byproduct of bacteria such as Lactobacillus and Lactococcus. These bacteria have been used for this property in combination with yeasts and molds in the preparation of fermented foods such as sauerkraut, cheese, soy sauce, pickles, wine, yogurt, and vinegar.

Antonie van Leeuwenhoek, a Dutch lens maker, was first to observe bacteria using a microscope he designed in 1683. His scientific observations were published in a series of reports to the Royal Society of London. Scientists were fascinated by his description of animalcules in human semen and pond water. Identification and study of bacteria did not begin until over a century had passed. Christian Gottfried Ehrenberg has been credited with being the scientist who introduced the word "bacterium" in 1828.

Louis Pasteur demonstrated in 1859 that the theory of spontaneous generation was incorrect. He also demonstrated that the fermentation process is caused by the growth of microorganisms, yeasts, and molds. Along with Robert Koch, Pasteur was an early advocate of the germ theory of disease. Koch was a scientific pioneer in the medical application of microbiology, and investigated the infectious causes of cholera, anthrax, tuberculosis and other life threatening conditions. Koch's research into the cause of tuberculosis proved that the germ theory was correct, for which he received Nobel Prize in 1905. Koch's postulates remain important scientific criteria to this day to prove that a specific organism is the cause of a disease.

By the nineteenth century, bacteria were known to be the cause of many diseases. Unfortunately, treatments for infections with antibiotics had yet to be developed, although there were some reports that moldy foods might be helpful. In 1910 Paul Ehrlich developed the first effective antibiotic by studying and modifying dyes that selectively stained the organism *Treponema pallidum*. This is the spirochete bacteria that causes syphilis, and a dye compound Ehrlich developed selectively killed the pathogen. Ehrlich received the 1908 Nobel Prize for his work on immunology and the use of various stains to identify bacteria.

Fungi

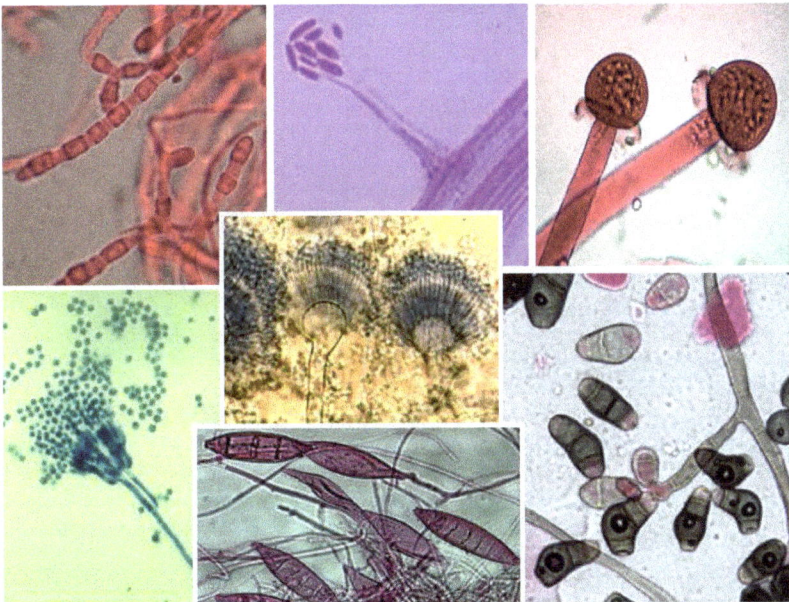

Collage of fungi. Public Health England

Fungi are eukaryotes and include yeasts, mold, mushrooms. Their cell walls contain chitin, not cellulose. The science of fungi is called mycology and was once considered a subsection of botany. Genetic studies have revealed that fungi are actually more closely related to animals than plants.

Parasite

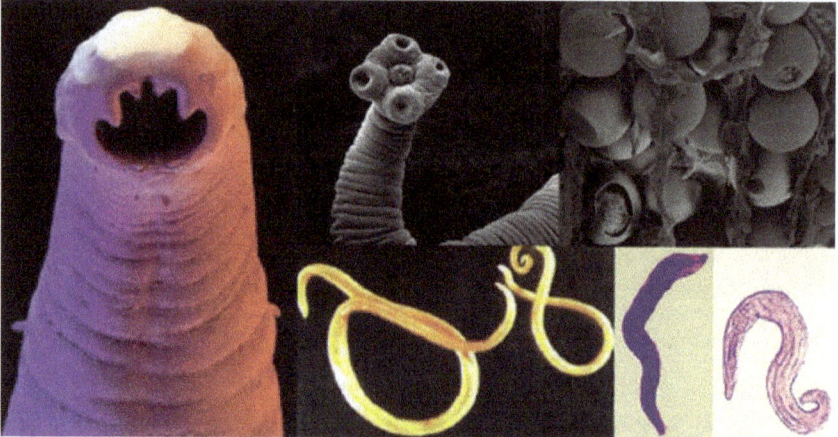

A variety of human parasites. Creative Commons License

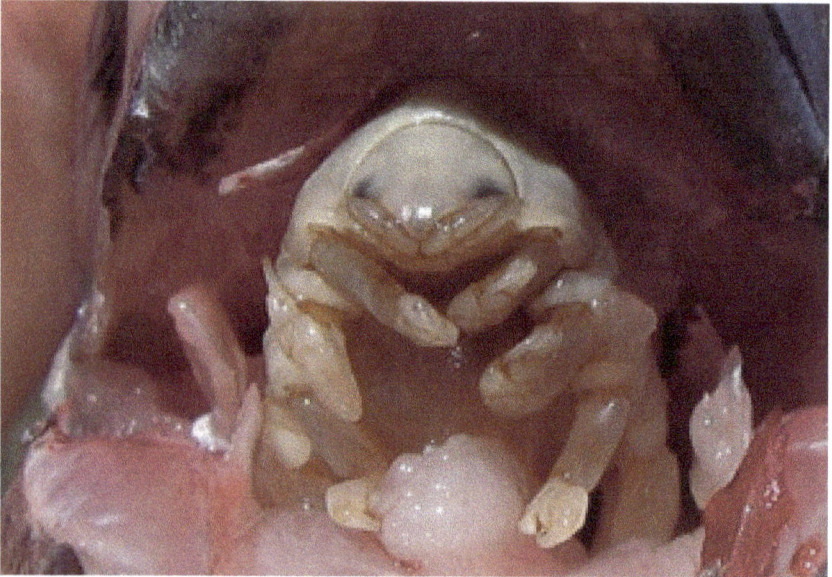

Fortunately for humans this nasty parasite is only found in fish. It eats the tongue of the fish and stays in its mouth ready to eat anything the fish consumes. Creative Commons License

Prion

Prions are fundamentally different than virus and contain and transmit infectious protein molecules that do not contain DNA or RNA. They can cause infections such as scrapie in sheep, bovine spongiform encephalopathy also known as mad cow disease in cattle, and chronic wasting disease in deer. In humans prion diseases include Kuru, which is acquired by cannibals eating the brain of a human infected with the virus. Other prion disease in humans includes Creutzfeldt–Jakob disease, and Gerstmann–Sträussler–Scheinker syndrome.

A prion is an infectious agent composed of protein in a misfolded form. The word prion was coined in 1982 by 1997 Nobel laureate Stanley B. Prusiner and is derived from the words protein and infection. Prions are responsible for the transmissible spongiform encephalopathies in a variety of mammals, including bovine spongiform encephalopathy also known as "mad cow disease". In humans, prions cause Creutzfeldt-Jakob Disease (CJD), Fatal Familial Insomnia, and kuru. All known prion diseases affect the structure of the brain or other neural tissue and all are currently untreatable and universally fatal.

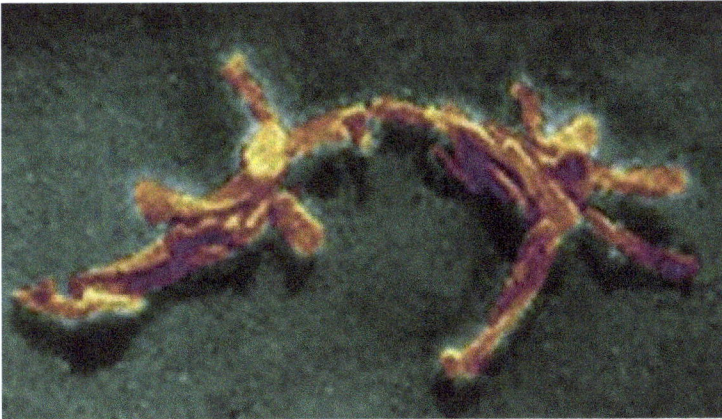

c0116801.cdn.cloudfiles.rackspacecloud.com Creative Commons License

Prions cause neurodegenerative disease by aggregating extracellularly within the central nervous system to form plaques known as amyloid, which disrupt the normal tissue structure. This disruption is characterized by "holes" in the tissue with resultant spongy architecture due to the vacuole formation in the neurons. Other histological changes include astrogliosis and the absence of an inflammatory reaction. While the incubation period for prion diseases is relatively long (5 to 20 years), once symptoms appear the disease progresses rapidly, leading to brain damage and death. Neurodegenerative symptoms can include convulsions, dementia, ataxia (balance and coordination dysfunction), and behavioral or personality changes. All known prion diseases, collectively called transmissible spongiform encephalopathies (TSEs), are untreatable and fatal.

Current research suggests that the primary method of infection in animals is through ingestion. It is thought that prions may be deposited in the environment through the remains of dead animals and via urine, saliva, and other body fluids. They may then linger in the soil by binding to clay and other minerals. A University of California research team led by Stanley Prusiner, has provided evidence for the theory that infection can occur from prions in manure. And since manure is present in many areas surrounding water reservoirs, as well as used on many crop fields, it raises the possibility of widespread transmission. Preliminary evidence supporting the notion that prions can be transmitted through use of urine-derived human menopausal gonadotropin, administered for the treatment of infertility, was published in 2011.

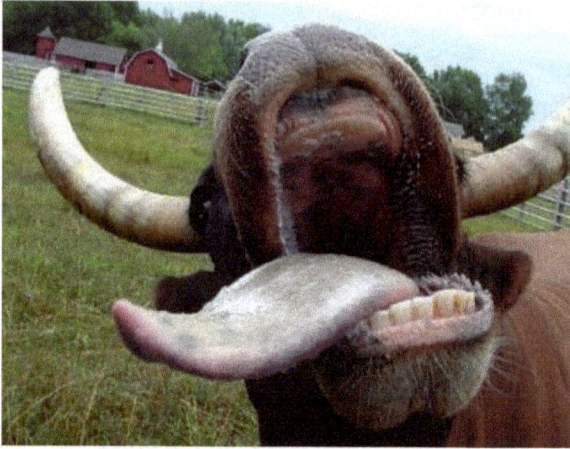

malialitman.files.wordpress.com Creative Commons License

Mad cow disease

Bovine spongiform encephalopathy, or mad cow disease, appears to cause a fatal human brain disease.

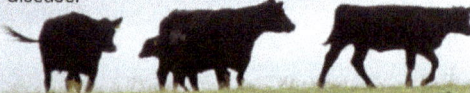

• **Severity** Cow begins "mad" seizures months or years after infection

• **Other livestock** Related disease called scrapie affects sheep

• **Prevention** Destroy infected farm animals; don't use animal products containing brain or central nervous system tissue as livestock feed

How it spreads **1** Person or animal eats food contaminated with brain or spinal cord tissue from infected animal

2 Disease attacks nervous system

Outer layer of brain develops tiny holes, looks spongy

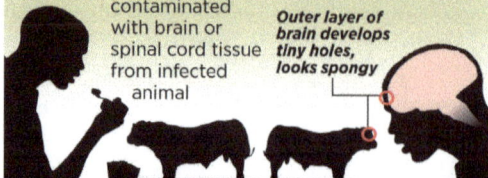

SOURCES: U.S. Centers for Disease Control and Prevention, U.S. Agriculture Department, MCT Photo Service

Creative Commons License

One of the recent illnesses identified as being caused by prions is mad cow disease also known as bovine spongiform encephalopathy. It is a fatal neurodegenerative disease in cattle that causes an encephalopathy characterized by a spongy degeneration of the brain and spinal cord. Bovine spongiform encephalopathy has a long incubation period from about 30 months to 8 years. It usually affects adult cattle at a peak age of onset of four to five years with all breeds being equally susceptible. In the United Kingdom, the country worst affected, more than 180,000 cattle have been infected and 4.4 million slaughtered during the eradication program. The disease may be transmitted to human beings by eating food contaminated with the brain, spinal cord or digestive tract of infected cattle. In humans it is known as new variant Creutzfeldt–Jakob disease and by 2010 had killed more than 200 humans. Up to 500,000 bovine spongiform encephalopathy infected animals had entered the human food chain before controls on high-risk offal were introduced in 1989.

The epizootic condition was caused by feeding cattle the remains of other cattle in the form of meat and bone meal, which caused the infectious agent to spread. The infectious agent is remarkable for the high temperatures at which it remains viable, over 600 degrees Celsius (about 1100 degrees Fahrenheit). The infectious agent in bovine spongiform encephalopathy is a specific type of misfolded protein called a prion. Prions are not destroyed even if the beef or material containing them is cooked or heat-treated. Prion proteins carry the disease between individuals and cause deterioration of the brain.

Transmission can occur when healthy animals come in contact with contaminated tissues from others with the disease. In the brain, these proteins cause native cellular prion protein to deform into the infectious state, which then goes on to deform further prion protein in an exponential cascade. This results in protein aggregates, which then form dense plaque fibers, leading to the microscopic appearance of "holes" in the brain, degeneration of physical and mental abilities, and ultimately death. Cattle are naturally herbivores eating grass in pastures. Modern industrial and commercial cattle farming use various feeds are which may contain additional ingredients and supplements including antibiotics, hormones, pesticides, fertilizers, and protein additives. Meat and bone meal from the leftovers of the slaughtering process as well as from the carcasses of sick and injured cattle or sheep was often used as a protein supplement in cattle feed in Europe prior to about 1987.

In order to control potential transmission of bovine spongiform encephalopathy related variant Creutzfeldt–Jakob disease within the United States the American Red Cross has established strict restrictions on individuals' eligibility to donate blood. Because of the very long incubation period individuals who have spent a cumulative time of 3 months or more in the United Kingdom between 1980 and 1996, or a cumulative time of 5 years or more from 1980 to present in any combination of countries in Europe, are prohibited from donating blood.

Cows affected by bovine spongiform encephalopathy show progressively deteriorating behavioral and neurological signs. One notable sign is an increase in aggression with cattle reacting excessively to noise or touch. With time the cattle become ataxic and may also develop a drop in milk production, anorexia and lethargy. At the slaughterhouse in the United Kingdom the brain, spinal cord, trigeminal ganglia, intestines, eyes and tonsils from cattle are classified as specified risk materials and must be disposed of appropriately without entering the human food chain.

In the US regulations prohibited the feeding of mammalian byproducts to ruminants such as cattle and goats since 1997. However byproducts of ruminants can still be legally fed to pets or other livestock, including pigs and poultry, such as chickens. The US Department of Agriculture (USDA) has recalled of beef supplies that involved the introduction of sick and dying downer cows into the food supply. Because the US standards and testing requirements are less rigorous than believed necessary to combat bovine spongiform encephalopathy many countries are hesitant to import its meat products. Sixty-five nations implemented full or partial restrictions on importing U.S. beef products. Beef consumption in the US was also affected by public concerns about food safety.

Protist

The protist are a eukaryotic microorganism that may be unicellular or multicellular and includes protozoa and amoeba.. A number of these organisms may be pathogenic to humans such as chlamydia, trichomonas, and giardia. The majority are considered commensals in that they do not harm nor do they provide benefit.

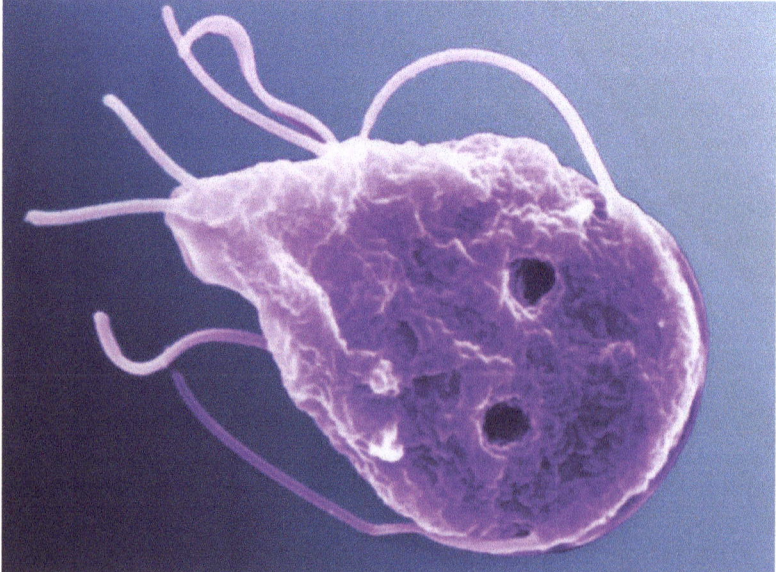

http://wellcomeimages.org/indexplus/obf_images/99/db/d408763f6cfcd8e0cc232c74db20.jpg
Giardia lamblia Creative Commons License

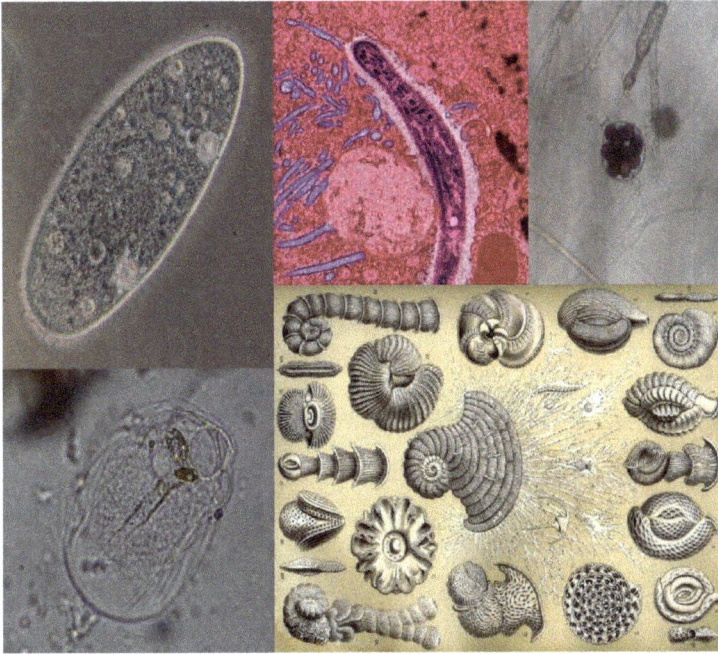

柑橘類 • Creative Commons License Protist collage

Virus

Virus (Latin virulentus poisonous) is a term that originally referred to poison and other noxious substances and was named by their discoverer Dmitri Ivanovsky in 1892. He mistakenly thought the illness transmitted from fluid filtered free of bacteria was a poisonous substance that the bacteria released. He did not realize that it was actually a living infectious agent much smaller than the bacteria that could not pass by the filter. Louis Pasteur was unsuccessful in his attempt to identify a bacterial cause for rabies. He speculated that the rabies pathogen may be too small to be seen using a microscope. In 1898 the Dutch microbiologist Martinus Beijerinck recognized that it was a new form of infectious agent but mistakenly thought that a virus was a liquid.

There is some controversy as to whether viruses should be considered a form of life, or nonliving organic structures that interact with living organisms. Some experts have described them as 'organisms at the edge of life' since they resemble organisms in that they possess genes, they evolve by the process of natural selection, and reproduce by creating multiple copies of their genetic code. Viruses have genes but they do not have the cellular structure that many define as the basic unit of life. Viruses do not have an independent metabolism and must invade a host cell to make new products and replicate. There are more viruses on Earth than stars in the universe. If you stacked every virus end to end they would stretch over one hundred thousand light years.

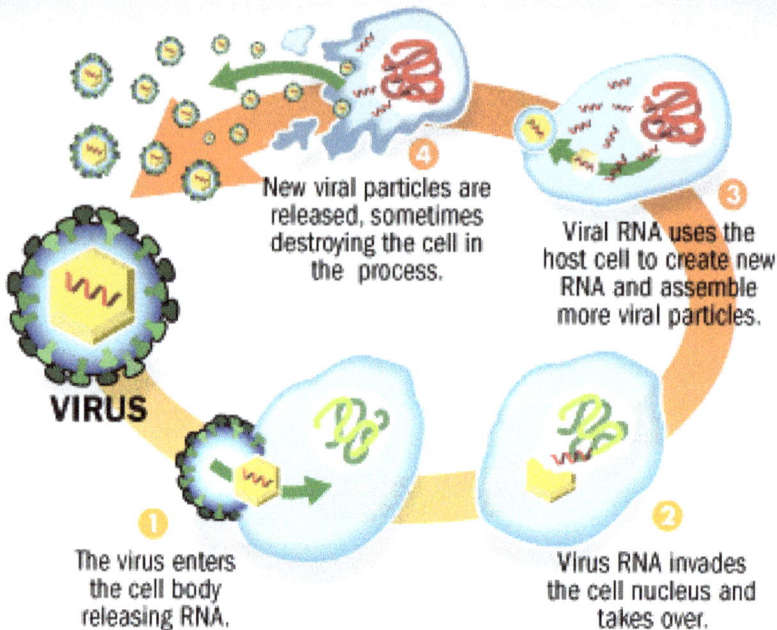

How a Virus Works
©2010 HowStuffWorks

4 New viral particles are released, sometimes destroying the cell in the process.

3 Viral RNA uses the host cell to create new RNA and assemble more viral particles.

VIRUS

1 The virus enters the cell body releasing RNA.

2 Virus RNA invades the cell nucleus and takes over.

Creative Commons License

A virion is a complete virus particle. It consists of the genetic material in the form of a nucleic acid that is enveloped by a protein protective coat called a capsid. The capsid is formed from the assembly of identical protein subunits, each of which is called a capsomere. Some viruses have a protective lipid envelope that was derived from the host cell membrane. The capsid is made from proteins, the nature of which are determined by the viral genome. The shape of the virion serves as the characteristic basis for the morphological distinction and classification of viruses. The shape can range from a simple helical structure to more complex structures such as an icosahedral forms. The average virus is only about one percent of the size of the average bacterium. Most viruses are so small that they cannot be seen directly with a standard optical microscope.

A very wide diversity of genomic structures can be seen among viral species. Viruses exhibit more genomic and structural diversity than bacteria, plants, Archaea, or animals. There are many millions of different types of viruses, yet to date only about five thousand have been described in detail. A virus may have either a DNA based or a RNA based genome, and is called a DNA virus or an RNA virus on this important distinction. The majority of viruses have RNA based genomes.

Viruses are the most numerous living organisms on Earth and they outnumber all of the other life forms combined. Viruses can infect all types of cellular life including plants, animals, fungi, and bacteria. Each specific type of viruses can infect only a limited range of hosts, and a number of viruses are species-specific. For example, the smallpox virus can infect only humans and it is therefore described as having a narrow host range. Other viruses that are described as having a broad range include the rabies virus, which can infect different species of mammals. The viruses that infect plants are nearly always harmless to animals. Most viruses that infect other animals are not pathogenic to humans.

Viruses may spread in a wide variety of ways including blood sucking insects and animals. When these animals or insects serve to transmit the disease bearing organisms they are known as vectors. Influenza viruses are spread through the aerosolization of the virions by coughing and sneezing. Norovirus and rotavirus are two of the most common causes of viral gastroenteritis and are transmitted by the fecal oral route. They are transmitted by direct contact or by entering the body through contaminated food or water.

A bacteriophage (Greek φαγεῖν*phagein* phage devour) is a virus that infects and replicates within bacteria. Bacteriophages consist of various proteins that envelope and encapsulate a DNA or RNA genome. The bacteriophage may have a relatively simple or an elaborate structure. The bacteriophage genome may be small and encode as few as four genes, or it may be very large and contain hundreds of genes. The bacteriophage genetic material is injected into the cytoplasm and replicates within the bacteria cell.

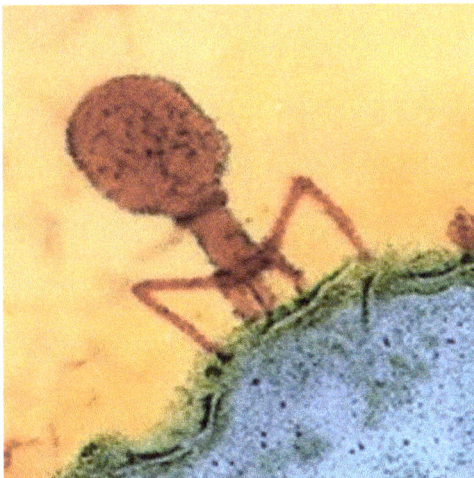

dennehylab.bio.qc.cuny.edu Creative Commons License

Bacteriophages are distributed widely and found in virtually all environments that harbor bacteria, such as soil or the gastrointestinal tracts of humans and animals. Seawater has one of the highest concentrations of bacteriophages in a natural nonliving environments. Bacteriophages and other viruses have a density in seawater of up to 9×10^8 virions per milliliter. These concentrations have been found in seawater microbial mats at the ocean surface. Up to seventy percent of marine bacteria may be infected by bacteriophages. Bacteriophages have also been used for over ninety years in the treatment of bacterial infections as an alternative to antibiotics in Russia, Central Europe, and France. Bacteriophages may have a role as a possible antimicrobial therapy against strains of bacteria that have developed resistance to many antibiotics.

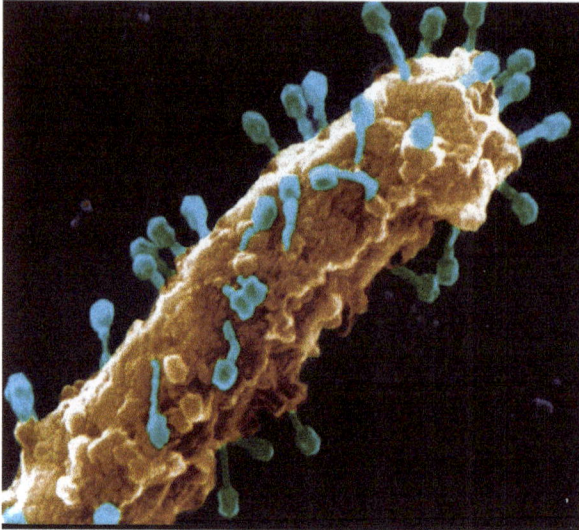

Swarm of bacteriophages attacking a bacterium rafefurst.files.wordpress.com Creative Commons License

Drinking the waters of various rivers as an effective treatment to cure infectious diseases has been documented since ancient times. In 1896, Ernest Hanbury Hankin reported that drinking the waters of the Ganges and Yamuna rivers in India could be effective in the treatment of cholera. The antibacterial action of the river water against cholera remained even if the water was passed through a very fine porcelain filter.

The antibacterial action was transmitted via the presence of microscopic viral bacteriophages in the river water. The discovery of the nature of viruses and their genetic structure and replication resulted in scientists Max Delbrück, Alfred Hershey and Salvador Luria being awarded the Nobel Prize in Physiology and Medicine in 1969. Bacteriophages are a very common and remarkably diverse group of viruses. In aquatic environments, they are the most abundant form of biological life comprising ninety percent of the biomass in the sea. In seawater they outnumber bacteria and Archaea by more than fifteen to one, reaching levels of two hundred and fifty million bacteriophages per milliliter of seawater. Most of the bacteriophages are harmless to plants and animals, yet are essential to the regulation of saltwater and freshwater ecosystems. It is estimated that viruses kill approximately twenty percent of the aquatic biomass each day.

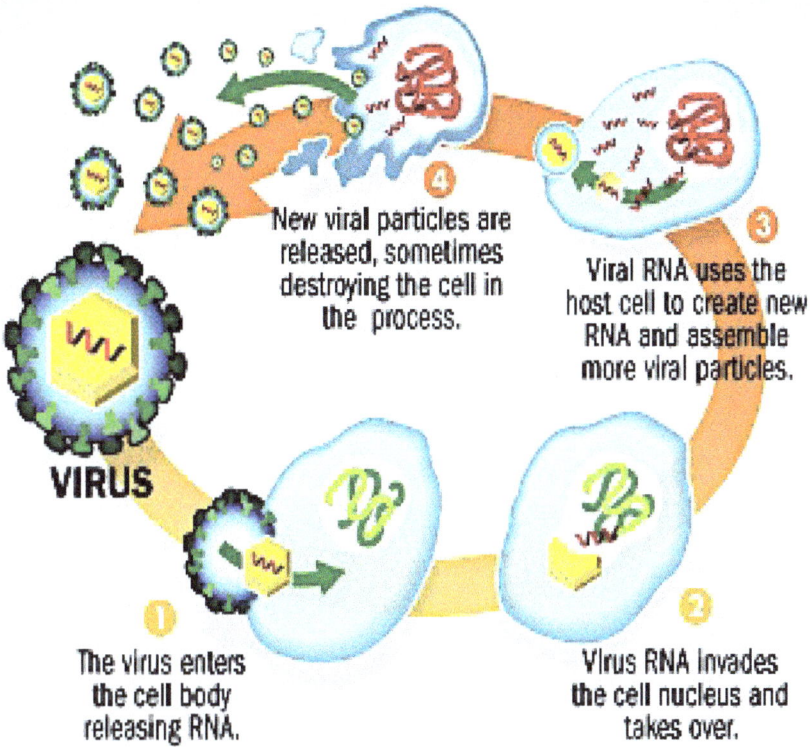

static.ddmcdn.com Creative Commons License

The bacteriophage viruses infect specific bacteria by binding to surface receptor molecules on the surface of the bacteria and then entering the cell. Within a short amount of time, often measured in minutes, bacterial polymerase starts translating viral mRNA into protein. These proteins may be new virions within the cell, helper proteins that assist in the production and assembly of new virions, or proteins involved in cell lysis. Viral enzymes may aid in the breakdown of the cell membrane. In the case of the T4 phage, overtaking the bacterial cell and producing and releasing over three hundred new virion phages could take place in less than twenty minutes from the time of infection.

Human immunodeficiency virus (HIV) is one of several viruses that may be transmitted via several bodily fluids, including through sexual contact and by exposure to infected blood. Antibiotics are not effective in the treatment of conditions caused by a virus viruses, but several antiviral drugs have been developed. Several examples of common human diseases caused by viruses include chickenpox, the common cold, and cold sores. And influenza. Viruses cause many serious diseases such as Ebola, AIDS, avian influenza, and SARS. The term virulence is used to describe the relative ability of viruses to cause disease. Some viruses can lead to chronic and even lifelong infections.

In chronic infections the virus is able to continue to survive and replicate in spite of the host defense mechanisms. This is seen commonly in untreated hepatitis B virus and hepatitis C virus infections. People chronically infected are known as carriers, and they can serve as an infectious reservoir for the virus to infect others. In populations where the proportion of the population that are carriers is high, the disease is said to be endemic.

Epidemiology is the area of science that deals with the study of health and disease in specific populations. Study of the transmission of viral infections in humans has demonstrated two different general categories. In the category of vertical transmission the virus is transferred from mother to child such as via the placenta or through breast milk. In horizontal transmission the virus is transmitted from person to person. An example of the vertical transmission of a virus occurs with the hepatitis B virus and HIV. With vertical transmission occurring in utero the baby has already been infected by the virus before it is born.

The most common form of the transmission of viruses in a given population is by means of horizontal transmission. Horizontal transmission can occur with the exchange of bodily fluids during sexual activity, blood transfusion, needle sharing, saliva from the mouth, etc. Horizontal transmission may also occur via contaminated food or water, aerosolized virions being inhaled, insect vectors such as mosquitoes, etc.

The incubation period, between the introduction of the virus to host and the first signs and symptoms of illness. Incubation periods are often of a characteristic duration for different viral diseases, and may range from a few days to weeks. The communicability period is the time when the infection can be passed from an infected individual or animal to another noninfected human or animal. It is during the communicability period that the illness is considered contagious. The knowledge of the length of time of both the incubation and communicability periods of specific viral infections is important in the control of outbreaks. An outbreak is described as an epidemic when there is an unusually high proportion of cases in a specific region, population, or community. A pandemic is the term used when the epidemic outbreaks occur on a worldwide basis.

Isolated populations that have not developed immunity to viruses can be decimated by epidemics. Among examples historically documented are the Native American populations that were devastated by contagious diseases. Smallpox was one of the infections brought to the Americas by European colonists that was particularly virulent in the native populations. The precise number of how many Native Americans were killed by infectious diseases after the arrival of Columbus in the Americas is not known, but numbered in the hundreds of thousands. It has been estimated that close to seventy percent of the indigenous population was destroyed. The decimation of the native population by diseases to which they had no natural immunity played a major role in the successful European colonization of native lands.

The catastrophic 1918 influenza pandemic lasted until 1919 and was caused by an extremely virulent and deadly influenza A virus. Unlike most influenza outbreaks that target the ill and elderly, most of the victims were healthy young adults. The influenza pandemic of 1918 may have killed as many as one hundred million people comprising five percent of the world's population at the time. The human immunodeficiency virus (HIV) is believed to have originated in primates in sub-Saharan Africa during the 20th century. HIV is a pandemic viral infection with approximately forty million people now living with the chronic disease worldwide. The United Nations and the World Health Organization (WHO) estimate that HIV has killed more than twenty five million people since it was first recognized in 1981. It has become one of the most devastating epidemics in recorded history, but has also led to research and therapeutic breakthroughs in the management of viral diseases.

Viruses are a known cause of cancer in humans and other species. Viral cancers can arise from both RNA and DNA viruses and occur in only a minority of infected persons (or animals). The risk of developing cancer is influenced by a number of factors including host immunity and genetic mutations. Viruses that are known to cause human cancers include several genotypes of the human papillomavirus, human T-lymphotropic virus, Epstein-Barr virus, hepatitis B virus, Kaposi's sarcoma-associated herpes virus, and the hepatitis C virus.

When the host immune system encounters a virus, it produces specific antibodies that bind to and inactivate the virus, making it non-infectious. This process is known as humoral immunity and is dependent two important classes of antibodies. The first class of antibodies are known as immunoglobulin M (IgM) and are effective at neutralizing viruses. Immunoglobulin M is produced by the cells of the immune system for only the first few weeks of an infection. The second class of antibody is called immunoglobulin G (IgG) and its production can be maintained as long as necessary. The presence of IgM antibody in the blood of the host indicates a recent acute infection, whereas IgG antibody indicates the infection occurred sometime in the past.

The host immune system second line of defense of is known as cell-mediated immunity and involves immune cells known as T cells. The host cells of the body display self-markers consisting of short fragments of their proteins on the cell surface that identify the cells as belonging to the host. A host cell infected with a virus may also display the foreign protein from the infecting virus, which may act as an antigen to stimulate the immune response and identify the cell as being infected. The immune system T cell mediated response recognizes the foreign viral fragment on the surface of the infected host cell. As the cell has been recognized as infected it is destroyed by killer T cells. The T-cells that identify the host cells as being infected by the specific virus proliferate and intensify the immune response to the virus. Macrophages are immune cells that are specialized at antigen recognition.

Interferon production is an important component of the host defense mechanism. Interferon stops viral reproduction by killing the infected cell and its close neighbors. Human immunodeficiency virus (HIV) is often able to successfully evade the immune system by frequently altering the sequence of the amino acid components of the proteins on the virion surface. With the antigenic markers on the cell surface changing regularly, the antibodies the body produced for earlier versions of the antigen are no longer effective.

Because viruses use the host cell metabolic pathways to replicate, drugs toxic to the pathway of viral replication are often toxic to all host cells as well. The most effective approach to controlling viral diseases are utilizing vaccinations to provide immunity, and the use of antiviral drugs that are able to selectively interfere with viral replication. Vaccination is an inexpensive and effective way of preventing infections by viruses. Their use has resulted in the significant decline in mortality and morbidity of serious viral infections such as mumps, smallpox, rubella, measles, and polio. Vaccines are commercially available for the prevention of over one dozen major viral infections of humans, and even more vaccines are available to prevent viral infections of animals such as livestock and pets.

Vaccines may consist of live but attenuated viruses, killed viruses, or antigens derived from viral proteins. Attenuated live vaccines contain forms of the virus that have been weakened to such a degree that they do not cause disease but can nonetheless confer immunity. Live vaccines have the potential of actually causing the disease they are meant to prevent, and can be particularly dangerous in causing active disease when given to people who are immuno-compromised. Antiviral drugs are often nonfunctional imitation analogues of the DNA nucleoside base building blocks. When a virus mistakenly incorporates a nonfunctioning analogue into its genome during replication, its life cycle is halted because the newly synthesized DNA is inactive.

Mountain Climbing (see Atmospheric Pressure, Ideal Gas Law)

Those who travel to higher altitudes, whether by climbing a mountain, driving up a mountain road, or traveling by air, experience an increase in flatulence. The underlying principle is the same, according to the gas laws of physics a reduction in atmospheric pressure results in an increase in the volume of intestinal gas. For those climbing hills and mountains with fellow travelers the incline usually means person behind has their nose at about the same level as the butt of the person in front. The practical take home message that is your advantage, if you understand the laws of physics, is to always be in the lead.

Another important consideration for those engaged in high altitude activities is the recognition that the oxygen content of air decreases with an increase in altitude. For those with underlying circulatory or lung conditions the additional stress of low oxygen content of the air can be potentially life threatening. Altitude sickness can also develop rapidly and is a life-threatening condition requiring an immediate descent in altitude.

Many air travelers are under the false impression that pressurization of the aircraft means the oxygen content of the air is the same as that on the ground at sea level. The aircraft is typically pressurized to maintain a cabin pressure equivalent to an altitude of approximately eight thousand feet. This leads to a reduction in the oxygen content of the air on the aircraft. Some normal individuals find this reduction in oxygen uncomfortable and develop headaches and other symptoms. Others are more sensitive, or recognize that their underlying medical condition requires that they have access to supplemental oxygen for their safe travel.

Nitrogen

Nitrogen is a chemical element with symbol N and atomic number seven is a colorless, odorless, tasteless, gas constituting seventy-eight percent by volume of Earth's atmosphere. The element nitrogen was discovered by Scottish physician Daniel Rutherford, in 1772. Nitrogen is the largest volume component of atmospheric air, and as would be expected, represents an identically high proportion of the gasses swallowed through aerophagia. Once in the body the carbon dioxide of the air is absorbed and eliminated as discussed above. The nitrogen however is a very poorly absorbed gas, and in essence will either come back up as a burp, or will sooner or later, comes out the other end as a fart.

The oxygen in the air, representing nearly twenty-one percent of the air gasses swallowed during aerophagia, is absorbed slowly, as the gut is not nearly as efficient as the lungs for respiration. As the carbon dioxide and oxygen are absorbed the percent of the gastrointestinal tract air that is nitrogen increases. As soon as the digestive process begins, hydrochloric acid of the stomach is neutralized by bicarbonate of the duodenum and pancreas. Large volumes of carbon dioxide gas are generated, as are smaller quantities of hydrogen, methane and other aromatic gasses discussed later.

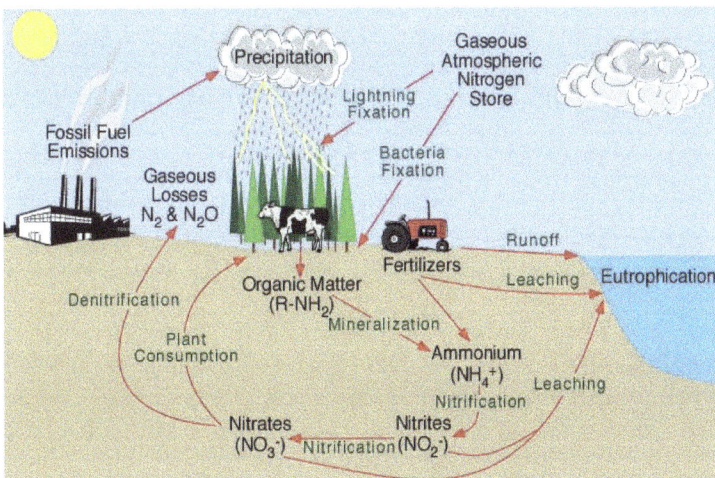

Pidwirny, M. "The Nitrogen Cycle" www.physicalgeography.net Creative Commons License

The nitrogen cycle is one of the most important nutrient cycles found in ecosystems. Living organisms use nitrogen in the production of complex organic molecules like amino acids, proteins, and nucleic acids. The nitrogen found in the atmosphere as a gas is about one million times larger than the nitrogen contained in living organisms. Nitrogen is often the most limiting nutrient for plant growth because most plants can only take up nitrogen in two solid forms: ammonium ion (NH_4^+) and the ion nitrate (NO_3^-). Animals receive the required nitrogen they need for metabolism, growth, and reproduction by the consumption of living or dead organic matter that contains material partially composed of nitrogen. The characteristic odor of animal flesh decay is caused by putrescence and cadaverine, which are breakdown products of the amino acids ornithine and lysine, respectively.

Nitrogen occurs in all organisms, primarily in amino acids, proteins, and in the nucleic acids DNA and RNA. The human body contains about three percent by weight of nitrogen, the fourth most abundant element in the body after oxygen, carbon, and hydrogen. It is a large component of animal waste (for example, guano) in the form of urea, uric acid, and ammonium compounds, which are valuable fertilizers. Nitrogen compounds were well known by the Middle Ages. Alchemists knew the mixture of nitric and hydrochloric acids, called aqua regia (royal water) could dissolve gold (the king of metals). Nitrogen compounds were used in saltpeter for gunpowder, and later as fertilizer. Nitrogen is used in beer due to the smaller bubbles it produces, which makes the beer smoother and headier.

When inhaled at pressures higher than four atmospheres nitrogen can act as an anesthetic agent causing nitrogen narcosis, a temporary semi-anesthetized state of mental impairment similar to that caused by nitrous oxide. Nitrogen also dissolves in the bloodstream and body fats. Rapid decompression (in the case of divers ascending too quickly, or astronauts decompressing too quickly can lead to life threatening decompression sickness (formerly known as caisson sickness or the bends), when nitrogen bubbles form in the bloodstream, nerves, joints.

Olestra

Olestra is a fat, cholesterol, and calorie free fat substitute that offers the mouth feel of fat without its nutritional consequences. It has been used in the preparation of otherwise high-fat content snack foods such as potato chips since it gained Food and Drug Administration (FDA) approval for use as a replacement for fats and oils in 1996. A popular olestra containing snack named Wow became the source of reports of gastrointestinal complaints including oily anal leakage and pungent intestinal gas. Subsequent studies suggested the gastrointestinal side effects might have been due to excessive intake of the product. Consumer concerns contributed to prohibition of the use or sale of olestra products in the European Union and Canada.

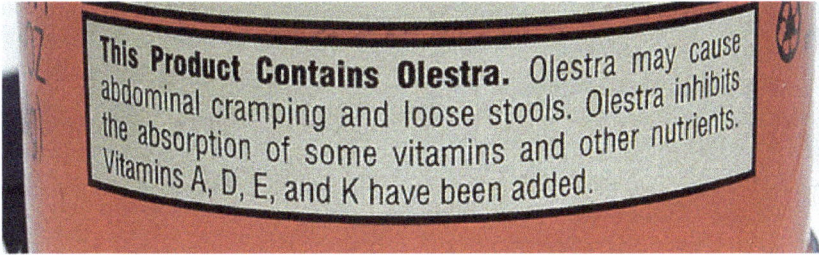

This Product Contains Olestra. Olestra may cause abdominal cramping and loose stools. Olestra inhibits the absorption of some vitamins and other nutrients. Vitamins A, D, E, and K have been added.

Triglycerides consist of three fatty acids bonded to glycerol, which acts as its backbone. Olestra uses the sugar sucrose as its backbone and bonds between six to eight fatty acids in a radial arrangement. This makes the molecule too irregular and too sizable to be absorbed by the intestinal lining, and it passes through the gut undigested. As it is not absorbed, it has no nutritive or caloric value. Because it contains fatty acids it can absorb and carry fat-soluble vitamins such as Vitamins A, D, E, and K with it as it transits the gut. Most products containing olestra are fortified with lipid soluble vitamins because of this effect, which could otherwise lead to malabsorption of these necessary nutrients.

Orlistat

Orlistat is a pharmaceutical designed to treat obesity. In the United States it is marketed as a prescription drug under the trade name Xenical, and is sold over-the-counter as Alli. Orlistat is a local inhibitor of gastric and pancreatic lipases and prevents the hydrolysis of triglycerides into absorbable free fatty acids. The triglycerides are excreted undigested in the feces along with the orlistat, which is not absorbed systemically. Taken three times daily before meals it prevents approximately 25% of dietary fat from being absorbed, resulting in modest weight loss in conjunction with a reduced calorie diet.

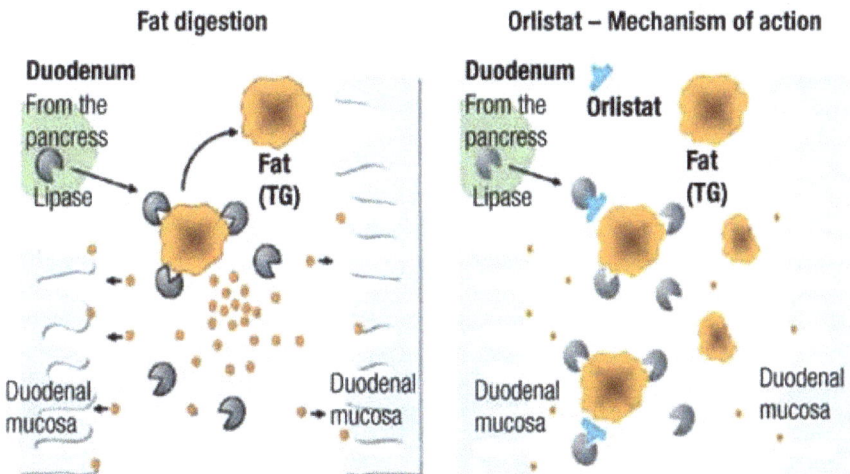

Orlistat – mechanism of action.
Creative Commons License

As expected with inhibition of fat absorption, Orlistat is notorious
for steatorrhea, oily, loose, and foul smelling stools. These decrease with time,
especially with the learned aversion of fatty foods, one of the behavioral
modifications that lead to the desired weight loss. Absorption of fat-
soluble vitamins and other fat-soluble nutrients are inhibited by the use of
orlistat. A multivitamin tablet containing vitamins A, D, E, K, and beta-
carotene should be taken once a day as a supplement when using orlistat.

Oxygen

Oxygen is a chemical element with symbol O and atomic number 8 that firms
dioxygen a colorless odorless, and tasteless gas. It was mistakenly named Oxygen
(the Greek ὀξύς (oxys) "acid", and γόνος (gonos) "producer"), by Antoine
Lavoisier who thought that all acids required oxygen (they require hydrogen). It
was discovered by Carl Scheele Sweden in 1773 but his publisher delayed
publication for two years. This inadvertently allowed British clergyman Joseph
Priestley, who independently discovered it a year later, to be given priority as its
discoverer because his work was published first.

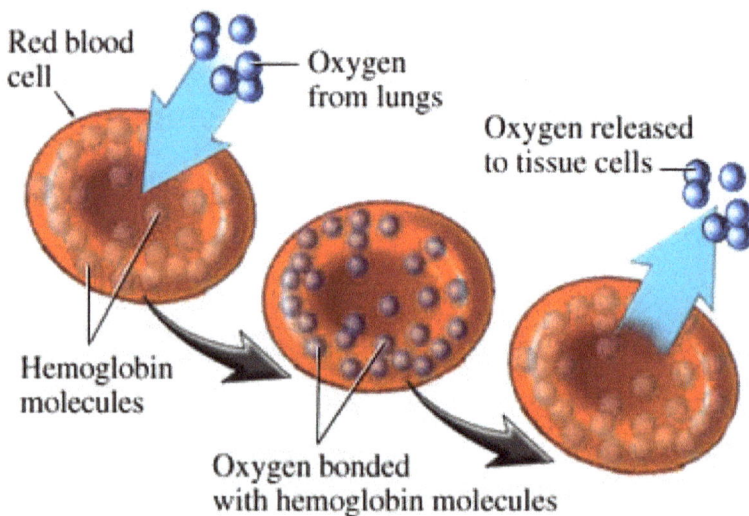

Red blood cell — Oxygen from lungs — Oxygen released to tissue cells — Hemoglobin molecules — Oxygen bonded with hemoglobin molecules

Oneminutecure.com Creative Commons License

Oxygen is a highly reactive element that forms compounds with most elements
except the noble gases. Oxygen is a strong oxidizing agent and only fluorine has
greater electronegativity. Oxygen is the third-most abundant element in the
universe, after hydrogen and helium. On Earth surface it is the most abundant
element making up half of the earth's crust, and makes up nearly twenty-one
percent of the air.

For free dioxygen to remain in Earth's atmosphere it needs to be replenished by the photosynthetic action of cyanobacteria, algae and plants. Free elemental O_2 only began to accumulate in the atmosphere about 2.5 billion years ago with the Great oxygenation event. Towards the end of the Carboniferous period 300 million years ago O_2 levels reached their highest levels of 35% and allowed insects to grow to a size with over a two-foot wingspan. I suspect that a mosquito that size would cause a human to pass out from blood loss if there were any humans to bite back then.

Cold water holds more dissolved O_2 which is the reason the polar waters support a much higher density of life then tropical waters.
The marine Cyanobacteria and green algae generate up to 70% of the free oxygen produced on Earth. In humans and vertebrates the O_2 changes the oxygen carrying hemoglobin to a bright red color. In mollusks and some arthropods like crabs hemocyanin gives a deep blue color when oxygenated. Hemocyanin uses copper, which has only one quarter of the oxygen carrying capacity as hemoglobin iron. If an iron nail is allowed to rust it will gain weight as it demonstrates its oxygen binding.

Parasite (see Microbiome)

Personalized Medicine

As with all issues of health and wellness each person needs to be assessed individually. With the advances in the human genome project it is now recognized that it is not just the genetic blueprint in the DNA that makes up the individuals uniqueness. Although humans have approximately 23,000 genes these genes are also controlled by external factors in a process described as epigenetics. It is also now recognized that the human body is in essence more than just human cells. The human system includes the microbiome, the microorganisms that live on and within us. The gut-brain-microbiome-food axis demonstrates the intimate interconnectivity of these four elements. If one were to analyze the human system by the number of cells a human is comprised of approximately 10% human cells and 90% microbial cells. If one were to analyze the system on the basis of the number of genes, humans are approximately 1% human genes and 99% microbial jeans.

The era of personalized medicine will advance the understanding of both health and disease. The previous approach of using population-based medicine will be abandoned as technology and bioinformatics allows treatments to be specifically tailored to the individual's genome, microbiome, and metabolome. The effectiveness of therapy should increase dramatically along with a significant reduction in adverse reactions to medications. This approach will also avoid the time and monetary expense of medications that did not provide a benefit, even if fortunately they did not cause an adverse reaction. In the interval as these advances are being brought into clinical practice it remains the best approach to tailor the treatment plan to the individual. What works for one may not work for another. Until the science and technology sufficiently evolve it often takes a trial and error approach to find the best treatment approach for the individual. And it is the individual who can be the only judge if the treatment is successful or the search for a solution must continue.

Physics

The laws and principles of physics apply to living as well as inanimate systems. An understanding of these principles explains many natural phenomena that are otherwise a source of mystery and confusion. When it comes to intestinal gas in particular, understanding the gas laws goes a long way in helping to manage this very common concern. Using Boyle's law, you can calculate how much the volume will compress as you go deeper underground or underwater. You can likewise calculate how much a gas will expand, as you go higher in altitude and the atmospheric pressure decreases. Using Charles Law you can calculate what happens to the gas in a cold drink when it is swallowed and is raised to body temperature

Boyle's Law

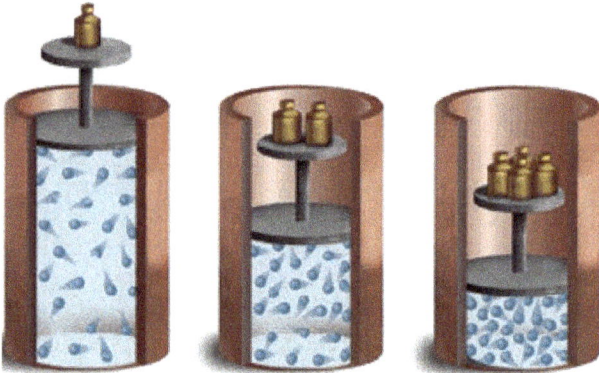

Charles's Law

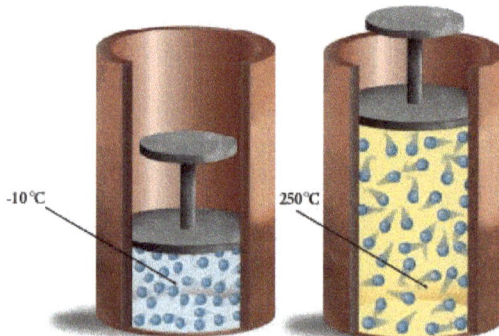

Creative Commons License

Prion (see Microbiome)

Protist (see Microbiome)

Rumination Syndrome

Rumination syndrome is an unusual condition and can lead to excessive air swallowing. Because the initiation of the rumination process itself requires the relaxation of the lower esophageal sphincter burps and belches are common findings. Rumination is typically seen in herbivorous livestock, which have compartmented stomachs to aid in the fermentation and digestion process. These animals regurgitate what is called the cud or partially digested food from the foregut stomach compartment to be chewed and swallowed again for further processes sings.

Humans can develop voluntary control of the esophageal musculature to retrieve stomach contents and swallow them again as if they were ruminant animals. The ability to train the esophageal muscles is most noted in yogi masters and circus performers but it is a learnable skill. Postprandial regurgitation is a symptom of rumination syndrome.

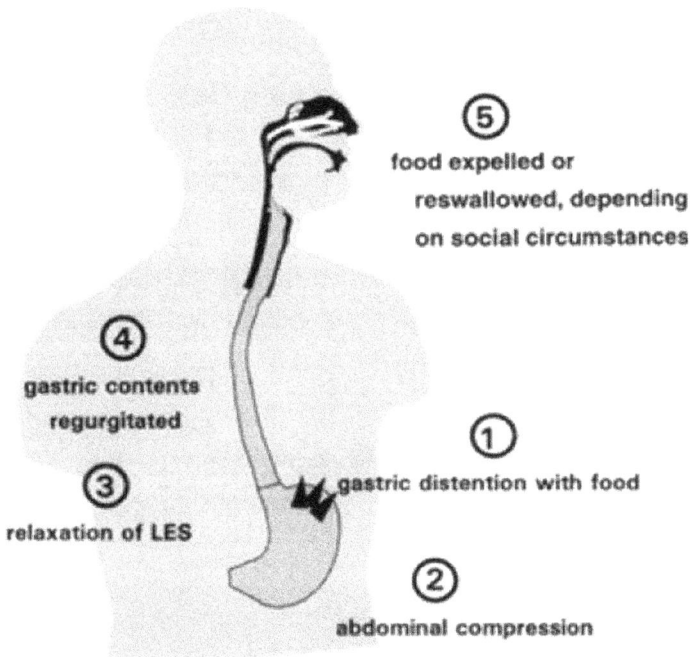

⑤ food expelled or reswallowed, depending on social circumstances

④ gastric contents regurgitated

③ relaxation of LES

① gastric distention with food

② abdominal compression

Rumination syndrome. Creative Commons License

For the others who subconsciously develop the rumination habit excessive air swallowing is simply the unavoidable result of the excessive swallowing that is part and parcel of the rumination syndrome. There are considerable psychological and psychiatric aspects of rumination disorders.

Scuba Diving (see Atmospheric Pressure, Ideal Gas Laws)

Scuba diving can be a very enjoyable activity, but it does require an understanding of the behavior of gasses and the laws of physics for safety. The atmospheric pressure changes associated with diving activity are pronounced and require close attention. Unfortunately, errors in judgment in scuba diving can be very unforgiving, and lead to fatal consequences if safety precautions are overlooked.

Boyle's Law was named after Robert Boyle, a chemist and physicist who published his discovery in 1662. The law describes that the pressure and volume of a gas are inversely proportional, if the temperature is kept constant. As the pressure on a gas increases its volume decreases, and vice versa, if you increase the volume of the gas, the pressure decreases.

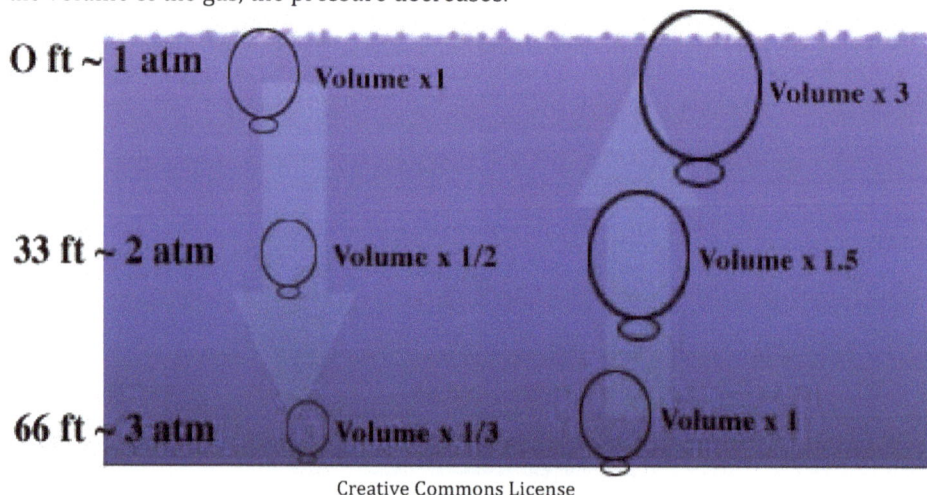

0 ft ~ 1 atm	Volume x1		Volume x 3
33 ft ~ 2 atm	Volume x 1/2		Volume x 1.5
66 ft ~ 3 atm	Volume x 1/3		Volume x 1

Creative Commons License

At the surface (0 feet) the pressure is 1 ATM (atmosphere). At a depth of 33 feet underwater the pressure is 2 ATM, the sum total of 1 ATM of air pressure and 1 ATM of water pressure. If a balloon with gas at the surface is submerged it will be one-half of the original volume at 33 feet depth, and one-third the volume at 66 feet depth. On ascent the balloon volume will be one and one-half times greater on going from 66 feet depth to 33 feet depth. It will have a volume three times greater at the surface than it did at 66 feet depth.

The diver experiences the effect of these pressure changes firsthand. As one descends the air in the facemask is compressed giving rise to the phenomenon known as mask squeeze. The pressure changes in the air spaces of the ear canal can be very significant if they are not purposefully equalized during descent and ascent. Severe ear injury including perforated or ruptured eardrum can result from unequaled air pressure. Head cold, allergies, sinus congestion, and other conditions that reduce the patency of the Eustachian tubes can prevent equalization of air pressure and should preclude diving activity.

The air volume in buoyancy control devices requires adjustment to maintain neutrality. The gas laws also explains why divers are advised to exhale while ascending as the gasses in the lung can over expand if the breath is held and result in severe internal injury. Dive bubbles increase in size as the gasses expand because of the reduced atmospheric pressure as they ascend. The gasses in the bubble are following the gas laws that dictate their behavior with changes in pressure, temperature and volume.

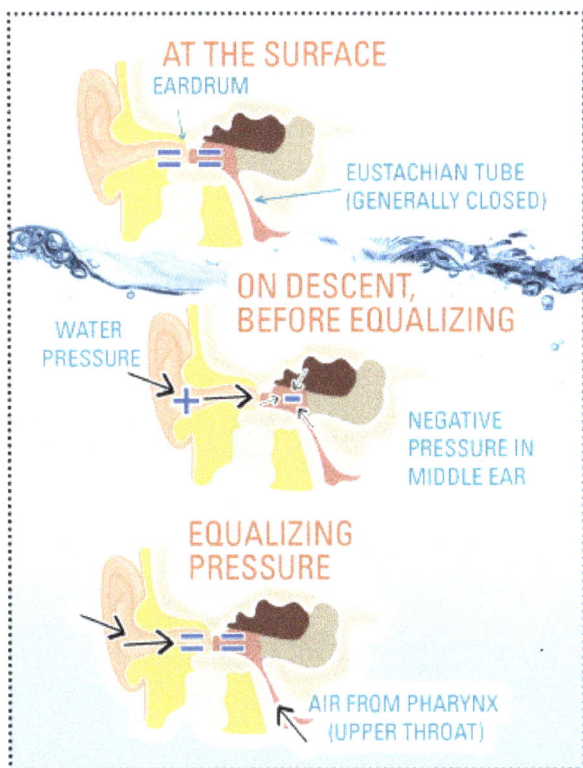

AT THE SURFACE
EARDRUM
EUSTACHIAN TUBE
(GENERALLY CLOSED)

ON DESCENT, BEFORE EQUALIZING
WATER PRESSURE
NEGATIVE PRESSURE IN MIDDLE EAR

EQUALIZING PRESSURE
AIR FROM PHARYNX (UPPER THROAT)

Creative Commons License

William Henry was an English physician and chemist who proposed what is now called Henry's law in 1803. The law states that at a constant temperature, the amount of a given gas dissolved in a liquid is directly proportional to the pressure of that gas. As the gas pressure increases, the solubility of the gas in the liquid increases. As the temperature increases, the solubility of gas in liquid decreases. The greater the pressure, the greater the quantity of a gas that can be absorbed by a liquid. The cooler the liquid, the greater the amount of gas that it can absorb. As the temperature of liquid increases, the solubility of the gas decreases forming bubbles that allow it to escape. Henry's Law explains why carbon dioxide in a pressurized container, such as in a can or bottle of a carbonated beverage remains in solution until it is opened. As soon as the container is opened the pressure is reduced causing the carbon dioxide gas to lose its solubility and escape in the form of bubbles or fizz.

In a similar manner as a diver descends nitrogen inhaled is under increasing pressure and becomes soluble in the bloodstream, muscles and tissues. This is not a problem until the diver begins an ascent and the pressure is reduced allowing the nitrogen in the body to form bubbles. If the diver ascends too quickly this can lead to Decompression Sickness also known as the bends. This is the reason why divers are advised to ascend gradually, to allow the nitrogen to be exhaled out of the lungs rather than to form bubbles in the bloodstream or tissue. Henry's Law also explains why after a dive the diver should not be exposed to higher temperatures such as a sauna, hot bath or shower or engages in strenuous activities or exercise. The increase in body temperature may cause the nitrogen to become less soluble and increase the risk of Decompression Sickness. Likewise diving in colder water enhances the absorption of nitrogen into the body, which should be adjusted for by shorter dive times or shallower dives.

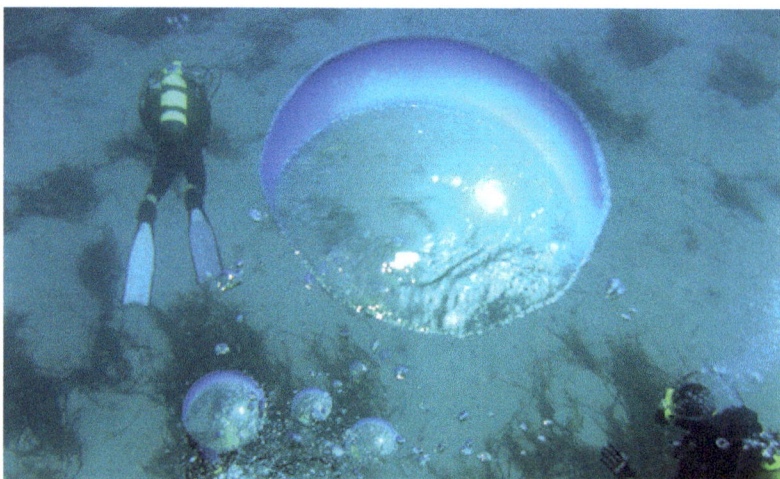

Creative Commons License

Charles' Law states that at a constant volume, the pressure of gas varies directly with the temperature. While a French philosopher named Joseph Louis Gay-Lussac published this law, Lussac attributed the law to an unpublished work by Jacques Charles. Jacques Alexander Charles was a French scientist, mathematician, inventor, and balloonist who studied the effects of temperature on the volumes of a gas. He formulated and published what became known as Charles' Law in 1787.

Charles wrote about the law after observing the effects of temperature on balloons. When a balloon is filled with gas and exposed to heat, the molecules of the gas cause the balloon to expand. When the balloon is exposed to colder temperatures, the molecules of the gas cause the balloon to deflate. The law states that at a constant pressure, the volume of a gas increases or decreases by the same factor as its temperature increases or decreases. Charles' law helps to explain the hazard of leaving scuba tanks out in the sun, or in the trunk of a car. The gas already under high pressure will have a further increase in pressure if subjected to heat, which can cause the tank to explode. The law also explains why scuba tanks increase in temperature when being filled with compressed air. Please see the entries on atmospheric pressure and ideal gas laws for more details.

Charles and Gay-Lussac's Law

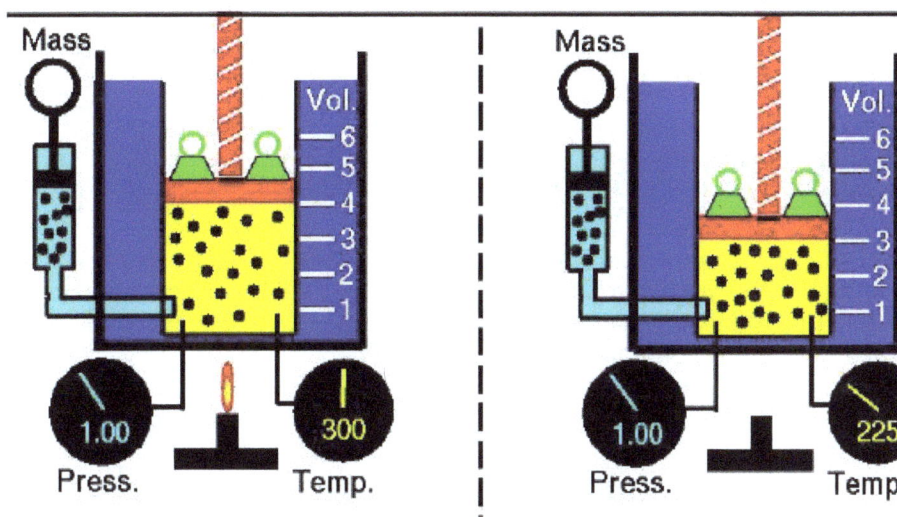

For a given mass, at constant pressure, the volume is directly proportional to the temperature

$$V = C\,T$$

Creative Commons License

Simethicone (see Bubbles, Surface Tension)

Simethicone is an oral over the counter product that is used as a treatment to reduce bloating, discomfort or pain caused by intestinal gas. Simethicone is a mixture of polydimethylsiloxane and hydrated silica gel, and is an anti-foaming agent that decreases the surface tension of gas bubbles. Surface tension is the property seen in water and other fluids that causes the formation of form semi-spherical droplets and bubbles. The reduction in surface tension does not eliminate the bubbles, nor does it cause them to become smaller.

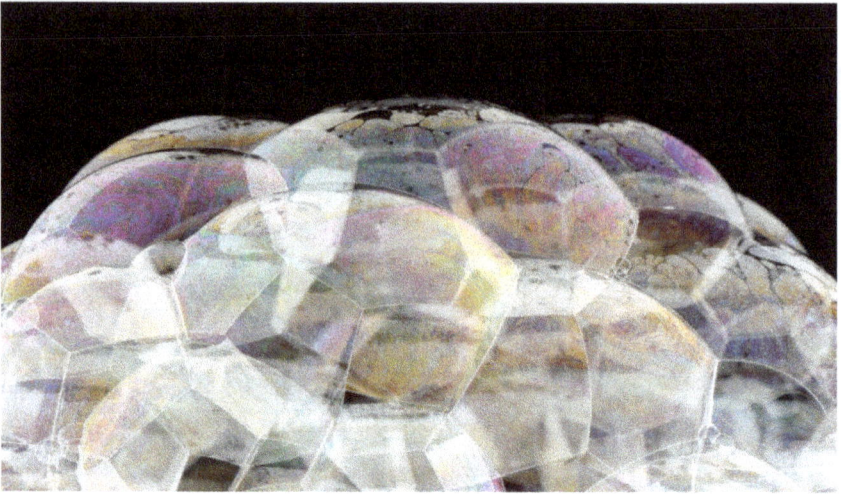

Creative Commons License

Counter intuitively, it actually causes them to combine into larger bubbles, and the presumptive relief is most often from being able to burp or belch up the larger bubble from the stomach more easily. There have been studies suggesting that simethicone increases the transit time so that intestinal gas may be more readily eliminated as flatus. Simethicone is not absorbed by the body and does not enter into the bloodstream.

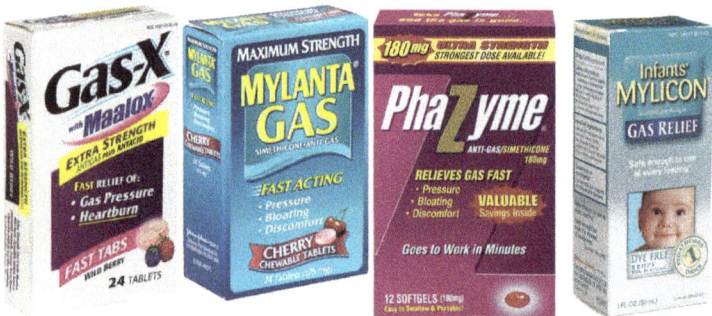

Creative Commons License

Simethicone has been promoted and marketed as a treatment for colic in babies, yet the actual cause of colic has yet to be clearly identified. Simethicone solutions of differing concentration also have industrial applications for reducing foaming in certain chemical processes, in detergents, as well as in medical imaging studies of the gastrointestinal tract.

Singultus (Hiccup)

Singultus, a hiccup, is an involuntary contraction of the diaphragm that may occur singly or in bouts. It is caused by a strong contraction, known as a myoclonic jerk, of the diaphragm. The diaphragm contraction increases the negative pressure in the chest cavity that cause the lungs to act as a vacuum inhaling a deep breath. Within milliseconds the epiglottis and vocal cords abruptly close creating a hic sound and cutting off the flow of air. A hiccup is an onomatopoeia, a word that was created to imitate the sound it is describing.

Hiccups are believed to be an evolutionary trait inherited from fish and tadpoles. The phrenic nerve which controls the diaphragm extends from the base of the skull and travels through the chest cavity. This design appears to have been derived from fish ancestors with gills closer to the neck. Interestingly enough as the human embryo develops the vestigial gills can be easily identified. The hiccup itself may have arisen from our evolution through the amphibian phase. The characteristic pattern of muscle and nerve activity of hiccups occurs in tadpoles that use both lungs and gills to breathe. When tadpoles use their gills they shut the glottis to close off the breathing tube while sharply inspiring. In essence tadpoles breathe with their gills using an extended form of a hiccup.

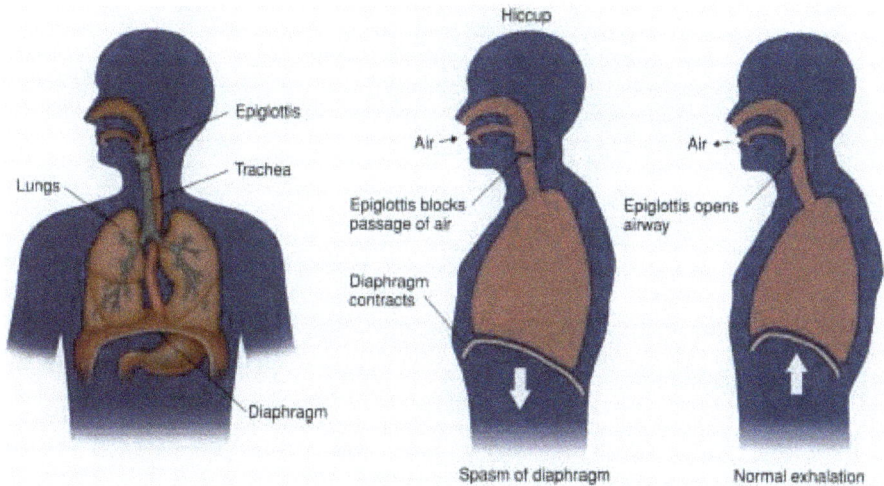

Creative Commons License

They resolve spontaneously in the vast majority of cases yet dozens of home and medical remedies exist that are not particularly effective. A recent theory proposes that hiccups developed as a reflex to allow the escape of swallowed air from the stomach during the suckling and feeding of infants. Pope Pius XII was seriously ill with a hiatal hernia and virtually uncontrollable hiccups in 1954.

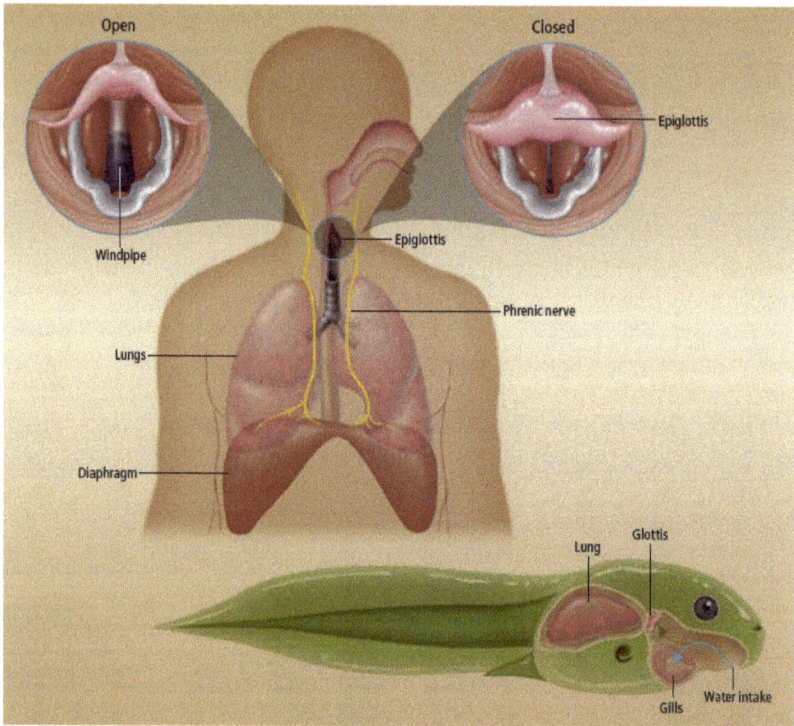

Creative Commons License

Common home remedies include: holding one's breath and exhaling slowly, holding the nose, breathing into a paper bag, sucking on ice cubes or hard candy, drinking water from the far side of a glass, gargling, pulling on the tongue, biting on a lemon, swallowing granulated sugar, swallowing hard bread crust, sneezing, peeling onions, bending over so that the head is lower than the chest, frightening the person with hiccups, slapping the person with hiccups on the back.

Spelunking

Spelunking, the exploration of caves, has become an increasingly popular activity and can take place above or below sea level altitudes. Some of the deepest explored caves have vertical drops in excess of one thousand feet. Although changes in atmospheric pressure are noticeable, this effect is one of the least dangerous aspects of the sport activity. The exploration of underwater caves known as cave diving, combines spelunking with scuba diving, and is a particularly demanding and challenging activity. In this activity understanding the potential effects of atmospheric pressure changes becomes critically important.

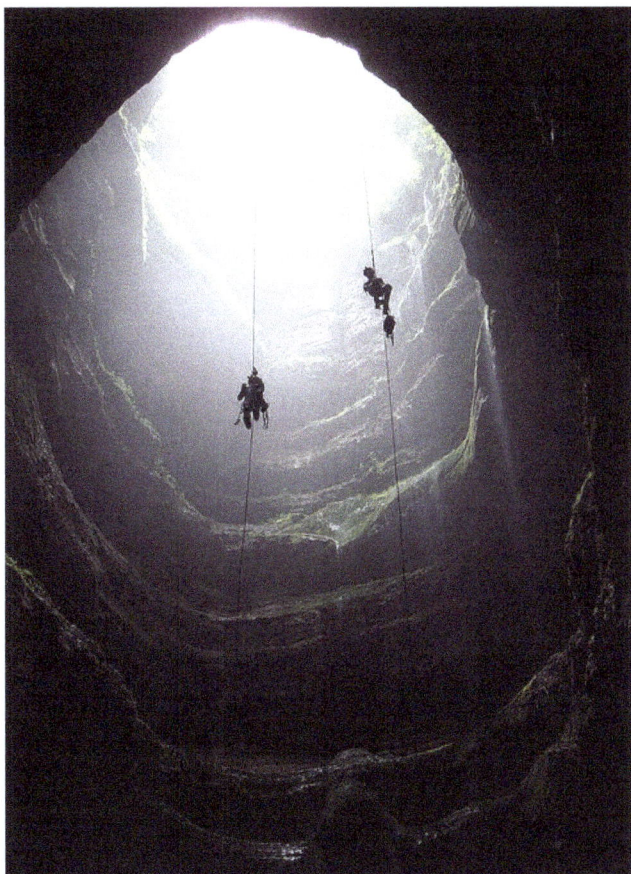

41.media.tumblr.com Creative Commons License

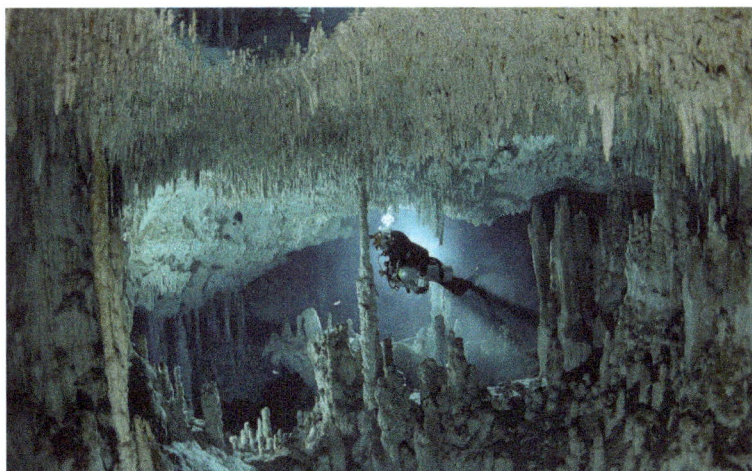

Creative Commons License

Surface Tension

Surface tension is a physical property exhibited when certain liquids are in contact with a gas. It is particularly pronounced when liquid water is in contact with the gasses of the air. Each water molecule contains two hydrogen atoms and one oxygen atom, giving rise to its familiar chemical shorthand of H2O. Because of their atomic structure the negative charge of the electrons of the hydrogen atoms are attracted to the positive charge of the oxygen atom, creating was is known as a hydrogen bond. The electric charges also create an attractive force between water molecules, causing them to want to remain close together. These forces are balanced out when a water molecule is surrounded by other water molecules.

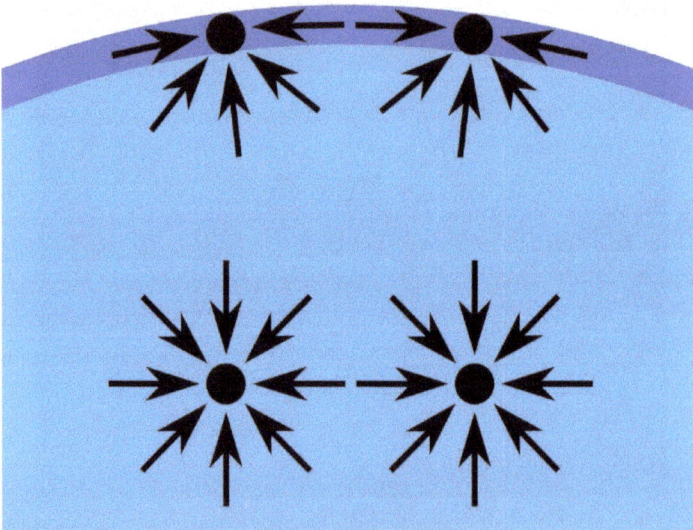

Booyabazooka Unbalanced charges on water molecules at the surface of a liquid gas interface.
Creative Commons License

When the water molecules on the surface are exposed to the gasses of the air above them they are no longer exposed to balanced charges. The water molecule on the surface exposed to the air is only subject to the electric charge pulling it down, keeping it in the liquid. This resistance to leaving its fellow water molecules behind gives it the property known as surface tension, a tension that prevents it from being separated from the remaining liquid. This surface tension is visible when you see water assume the shape of a droplet, or when you fill a glass to the brim and the fluid builds up above the lip of the glass before it begins to overflow. It is also the principle that allows insects heavier than water, such as the water glider, appear to walk on water because the surface tension acts as a walk able surface. Surface tension also is the force that allows the creation of bubbles. Surfactants are products that have the property of reducing surface tension and are used in detergents, as well as in anti-bubble and anti-gas products such as simethicone.

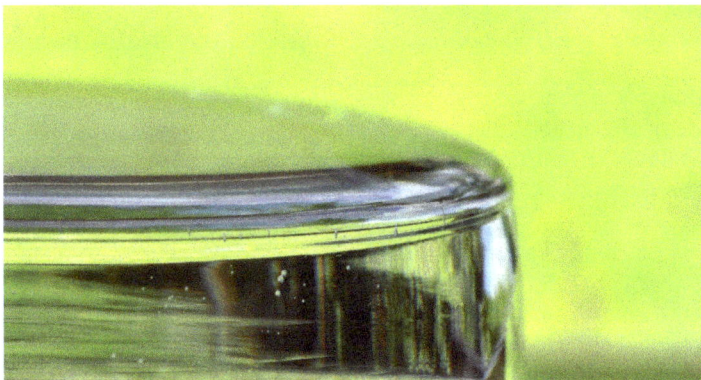

Surface tension allowing to go over brim of glass without spilling. Andre Roberto Doreto Santos www.flickr.com Creative Commons License

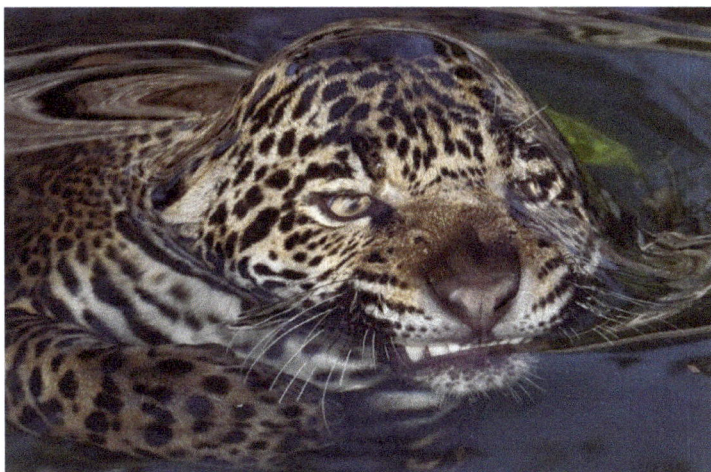

Photograph of surface tension effect. i.imgur.com Creative Commons License

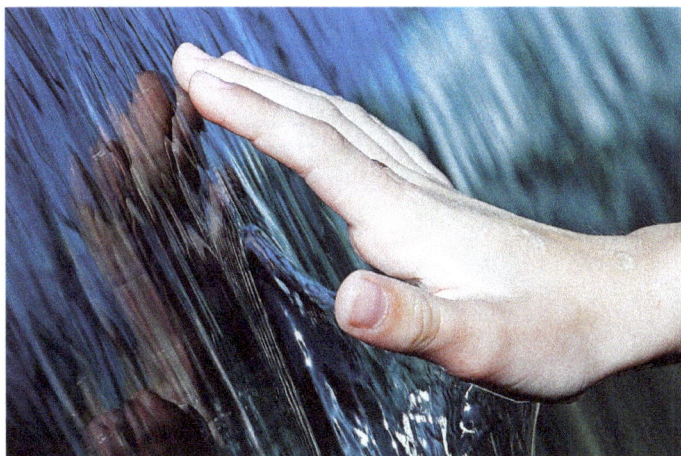

Photograph of surface tension effect. upload.wikimedia.org Creative Commons License

Underground Miners (see Atmospheric Pressure and Ideal Gas Laws)

Underground mining has significant occupational hazards. Some mines are subjected to pressurization to prevent the seepage of ground water into the mine. In other instances the mining activity may expose pockets of toxic gasses that can lead to injury or death. For those engaged in spelunking, the exploring of caves, descending to depths within the earth have hazards similar to mining related to atmospheric pressure changes. An understanding of the effects and dangers of changes in atmospheric pressure is critical to mine and cave exploration safety. Please see the entries on atmospheric pressure and ideal gas laws for further details.

Vagina (see Fart, Vagina)

Virus (see Microbiome)

Whoopee Cushion

A whoopee cushion is a device used as a practical joke which mimics the sound of flatulence when compressed. It is commonly placed on a chair or cushion so that the sound is generated when someone sits on it. It is typically constructed as a rubber bladder, which is inflated with air. A vibrating exit flap creates an audible fart like sound that is generated when sat upon. The modern commercially successful version was developed in the 1920's by the JEM Rubber Co. of Toronto, Canada. A more discrete alternate remote controlled version that can be hidden under a chair electronically generates prerecorded fart sounds

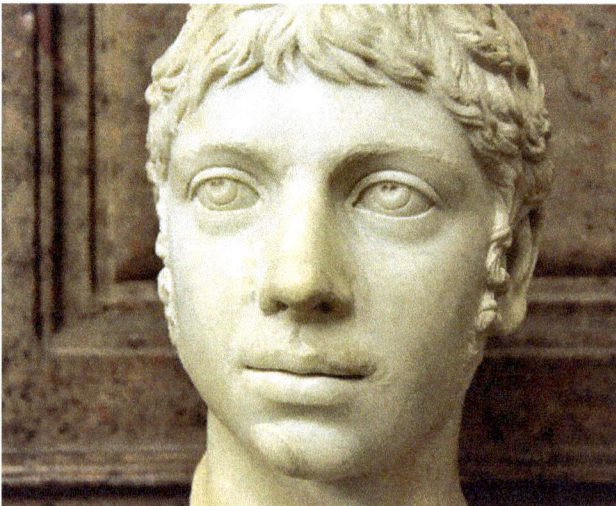

Elagabalus, Public Domain

Elagabalus, Marcus Aurelius Antoninus Augustus, (c. 203 AD – 222 AD) was Roman Emperor from 218 to 222. According to the findings of archeologist

Warwick Ball the Roman Emperor Elagabalus played practical jokes on his guests. At dinner parties he would place whoopee cushion like devices under their seats from which fart like sounds would emanate. He showed a disregard for Roman traditions and taboos, insulted the Roman Senate, the common people, and his own protectors the Praetorian Guard. It is therefore not terribly surprising that he was assassinated at age eighteen.

Yoga

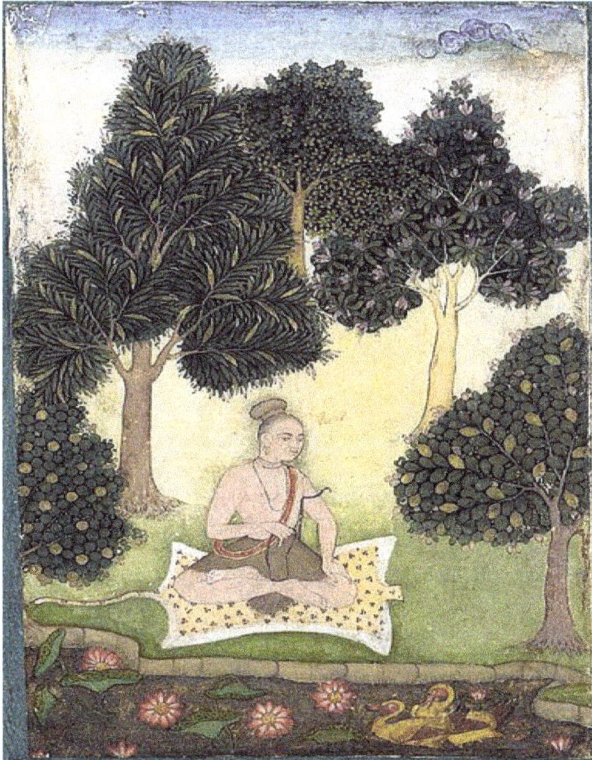

A yogi seated in a garden, North Indian or Deccani miniature painting, c. 1620-40
www.columbia.edu/itc Public Domain

Yoga is a physical, mental and spiritual practice that comprises many different schools and approaches. It has often been associated with the practice of Hinduism, Buddhism, Jainism and other belief systems that originated in the East. The origins of yoga are not clearly defined but were thought to arise in pre-Vedic Indian traditions. The first documents ascribed to yoga are found in the Buddhist Nikayas and the Yoga Sutras of Patanjali recorded around 400 AD. Recognizing its role in general health and wellness it is no longer an exclusive religious practice but has become increasingly adopted into the mainstream. Of course any general physical activity is beneficial as it increases bowel motility, yet there are a number of specific yoga postures that may provide additional benefit from compression and release of intra-abdominal pressure.

Yoga originally had been a religious practice and over thousands of years have become incorporated into secular wellness programs as well. Its effect on natural bodily functions, including intestinal gas were well recognized even in ancient times. Yogic masters and Brahmins in India practiced goze (flatus, eructation, belch) as a means of concentration in ridding the flesh of all evil. Yoga may provide benefit for some individuals with irritable bowel syndrome, especially poses that exercise the lower abdomen. It may also stimulate the passage of intestinal gas. In fact there is a specific yoga posture designed to aid in the release of intestinal gas. It is not unusual for participants in a yoga class to experience the auditory or olfactory consequences of someone else's, or their own, successful assumption of the yoga gas release pose.

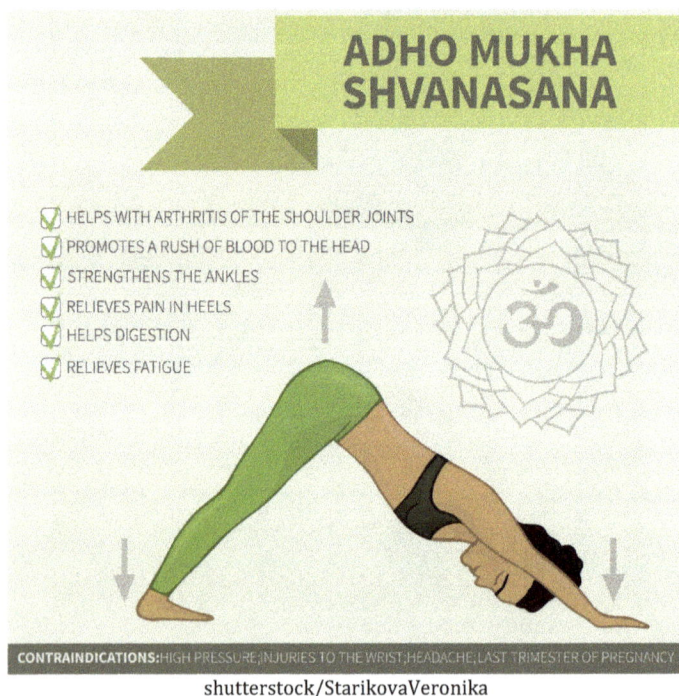

ADHO MUKHA SHVANASANA

- HELPS WITH ARTHRITIS OF THE SHOULDER JOINTS
- PROMOTES A RUSH OF BLOOD TO THE HEAD
- STRENGTHENS THE ANKLES
- RELIEVES PAIN IN HEELS
- HELPS DIGESTION
- RELIEVES FATIGUE

CONTRAINDICATIONS: HIGH PRESSURE; INJURIES TO THE WRIST; HEADACHE; LAST TRIMESTER OF PREGNANCY

shutterstock/StarikovaVeronika

It helped to achieving the suppression of consciousness and reaching towards enlightenment through union with the Supreme Being (Nirvana). Belching & forcing wind from the buttocks the yogi would chant: "Glory to those keen ebullitions which escape above & below!" (Allen Edwardes: The Jewel in the Lotus). Among certain Brahmins, a spiritual blessing was required after each bite of food: He takes a little rice soaked in melted butter and puts it into his mouth, saying: "Glory to the wind which dwells in the chest!' At the second mouthful, "Glory to the wind which dwells in the face!" At the third, "Glory to the wind which dwells in the throat!" At the fourth, "Glory to the wind which dwells in the whole body!" At the fifth, "Glory to those noisy ebullitions which escape above and below!" Any general physical activity is beneficial as it increases bowel motility, yet there are a number of yoga postures that may provide additional benefit from compression and release of intra-abdominal pressure.

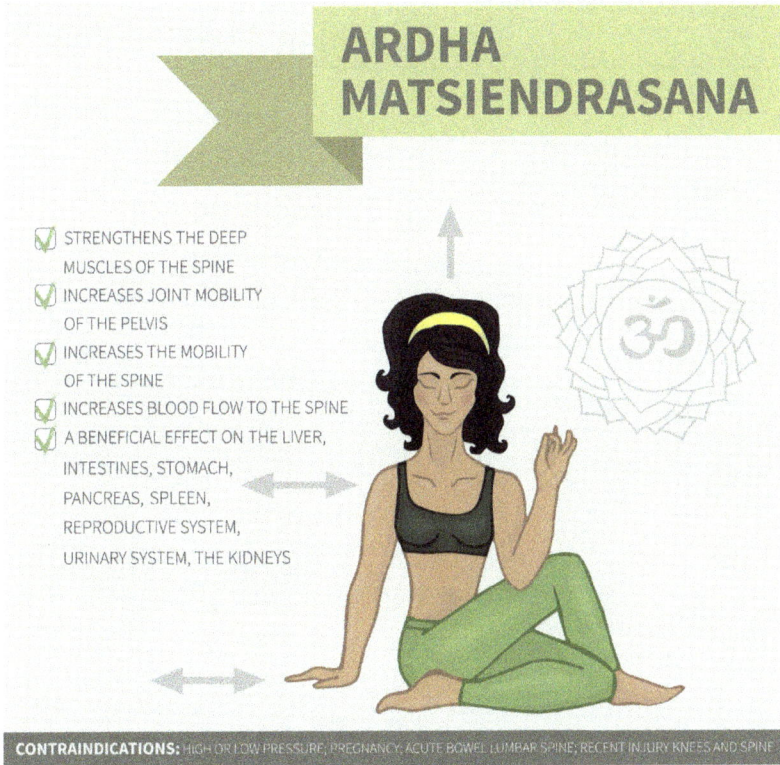

ARDHA MATSIENDRASANA

- STRENGTHENS THE DEEP MUSCLES OF THE SPINE
- INCREASES JOINT MOBILITY OF THE PELVIS
- INCREASES THE MOBILITY OF THE SPINE
- INCREASES BLOOD FLOW TO THE SPINE
- A BENEFICIAL EFFECT ON THE LIVER, INTESTINES, STOMACH, PANCREAS, SPLEEN, REPRODUCTIVE SYSTEM, URINARY SYSTEM, THE KIDNEYS

CONTRAINDICATIONS: HIGH OR LOW PRESSURE; PREGNANCY; ACUTE BOWEL LUMBAR SPINE; RECENT INJURY KNEES AND SPINE

shutterstock/StarikovaVeronika

The Wind-Relieving Pose (Pavanamuktasana) is particularly effective . (Sanskrit: Pavana wind, mukta relieve , Asana Posture) Technique: Lie on your back, arms by your side and feet together. Inhale and as you exhale bend your right knee and flex your right leg bringing the right thigh up pressing on the abdomen. Inhale again and as you exhale lift your head and chest up off the floor and touch your chin to your right knee. Hold this position for several more cycles of inspiration and expiration. Then relax and after a rest repeat the sets with the opposite side. After a second period of rest and relaxation repeat the exercises using both legs at the same time. Avoid practicing the Wind-Relieving Pose (Pavanamuktasana) if you have high blood pressure, heart problems, excess acidity reflux or GERD, hernia, slip disc, neck or back problems, or are pregnant or if you feel any ill effects from the exercise. Other yoga positions and moves that may be helpful include Balasana (Child's Pose) supported, Paschimottanasana (Seated Forward Bend), Supta Baddha Konasana (Reclining Bound Angle Pose) supported, Janu Sirsasana (Head of the Knee Pose) supported, and Jathara Parivartanasana (Revolved Abdomen Pose).

Sthala Basti, also called Vata Basti, Air Basti, Air Enema, is an advanced Hatha yoga technique that is best learned from an expert teacher. There are a number of different approaches and techniques but mastery of anal sphincter is a challenging practice. Once you master this technique you may not become as famous as the Petomane of the Moulin Rouge but you will certainly be able to entertain your soon to be former friends.

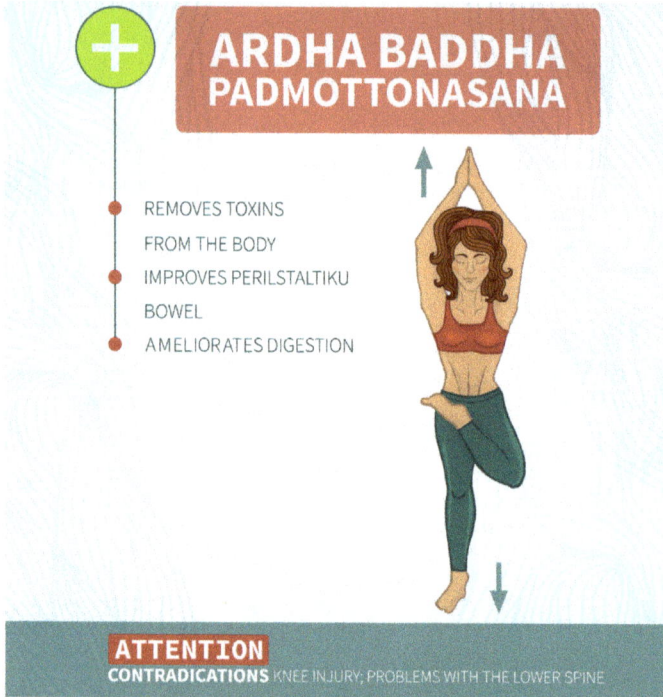

ARDHA BADDHA PADMOTTONASANA

- REMOVES TOXINS FROM THE BODY
- IMPROVES PERILSTALTIKU BOWEL
- AMELIORATES DIGESTION

ATTENTION
CONTRADICATIONS KNEE INJURY; PROBLEMS WITH THE LOWER SPINE

shutterstock/StarikovaVeronika

Sthala Basti starting from Paschimottanasana technique. Sit with your legs stretched out in front of you and then bend forward halfway. You do not however fully place your upper body on your legs but only bend forward halfway. Perform Uddiyana Bandha by exhaling completely then taking a false inhalation while holding the breath. This flattens and pulls in the abdomen under the rib cage as if the chest was suctioning it. The process is repeated many times followed by relaxation of the anal sphincter muscles to allow air to be drawn in with the uddiyanna Bandha maneuver. The air suctioned in is released as flatus.

Sthala Basti in lying Position technique. Lying on the back bend the knees up towards the chest and raise the buttocks. Practice developing control of the anal sphincter muscles by contraction and relaxation of the sphincter. When the sphincter is relaxed air suctioned into the colon is released as flatulence.

Sthala Basti in Utkatasana technique. Sit in Utkatasana, also called the chair or lightning bolt pose, by squatting while standing with the knees bent 90 degrees backwards to thighs. The back and upright arms form a forward facing 90-degree angle from the thighs. If necessary until sphincter control is mastered a hollow tube like bamboo or a catheter is placed in the anus and Uddiyama Bandha is performed. Air is sucked into the colon and released as flatus.

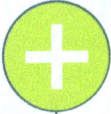

UTTANASANA

- STIMULATES THE KIDNEYS AND LIVER
- LOOSENS THE PELVIS AND THE CALF MUSCLES
- STRETCHES THE BACK OF THE THIGHS
- PULLS THE SPINE
- IMPROVES DIGESTION

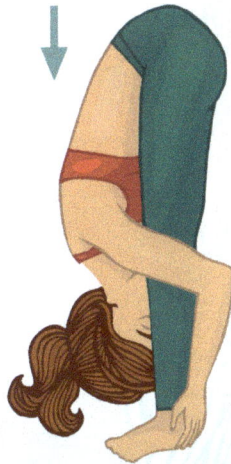

ATTENTION
CONTRADICATIONS HIGH AND LOW BLOOD PRESSURE; CIRCULATORY DISORDERS OF THE HEAD

shutterstock/StarikovaVeronika

Afterword

To 'Air' is Human, Everything You Ever Wanted to Know About Intestinal Gas
covers everything you ever wanted to know about the burp, belch, bloat, fart and
everything digestive, but were either too afraid or too embarrassed to ask. It has a
companion volume: ***Artsy Fartsy, Cultural History of the Fart*** is a fascinating
and factually correct review of the common fart through human culture and
history. The cough, sneeze, hiccup, stomach rumble, burp, belch, and other bodily
sounds simply cannot compete with the notoriety of the fart. Whether
encountered live and in person or through the medium of literature, television,
film, art, or music it may leave a powerful and lingering memory. The intent of the
book is to demonstrate that the ubiquitous fart has a more illustrious story to
share than just lowbrow humor. The societal standards and cultural acceptance of
this normal physiologic event have evolved over the years, and it is currently
popular as a point of humor even in sophisticated circles. The history of the fart in
culture and society is a seldom told but fascinating tale.

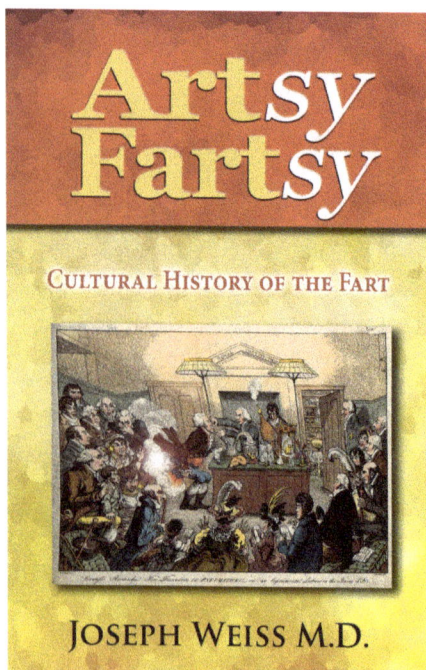

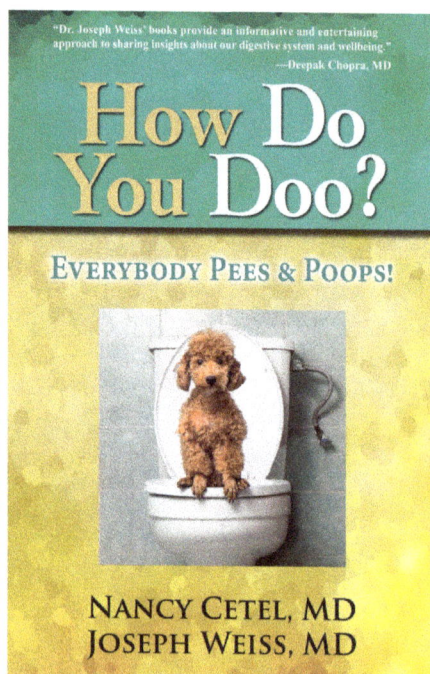

How Do You Doo? Everybody Pees & Poops! A delightfully informative,
entertaining, and colorfully illustrated volume with valuable practical insights on
toilet training. Tasteful color photographs of animals answering the call of nature
allows the child to understand that everybody does it! Additional informative
relevant content to entertain the adult while the child is 'on the potty' is included.

The Scoop on Poop! Flush with Knowledge is a uniquely informative tastefully entertaining, and well-illustrated volume that is full of it! The 'it' being a comprehensive and knowledgeable overview of all topics related to the remains of the digestive process. Whether you call it poop, feces, excrement, manure, dung, or the hundred plus other euphemisms, shit happens, and it happens a lot! Tens of billions of pounds and kilograms of it or deposited every day by while diversity of animal and microbial life. Humans alone contribute over three billion pounds a day, and only a small percentage of that is treated by a sewage system

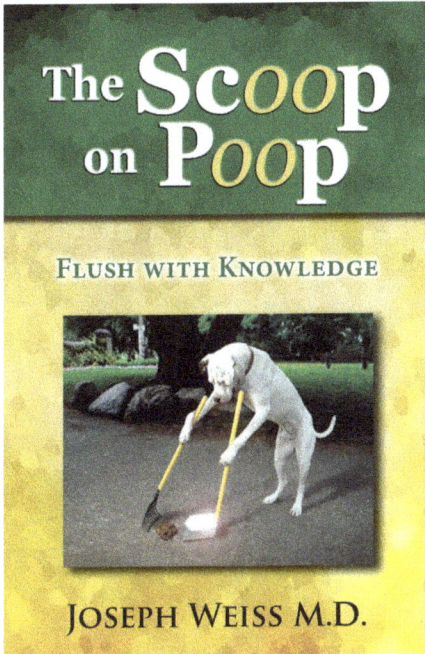

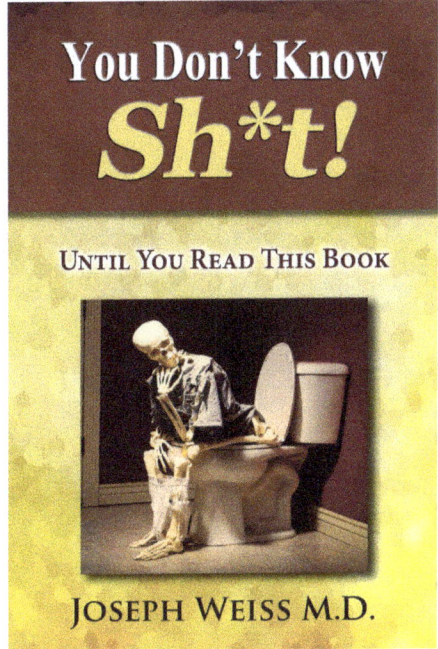

The identical content of The Scoop on Poop has been provocatively and cheekily retitled as ***You Don't Know Sh*t! Until You Read This Book***. This volume is an informative, entertaining and colorfully illustrated fountain of knowledge that is full of valuable information, including eccentricities and peculiarities, about the remains of the digestive process. Although this end result is politely described as feces or excrement, it is more commonly known by one of oldest words in the English language, shit. The book covers everything you ever wanted to know about this subject. Whether you disdain it, or appreciate it, it is part of the human (and animal) experience. The purpose of this volume is to share rarely discussed but very important knowledge about poop. The information ranges from the potentially life-saving to the sidesplitting descriptions of the eccentricities and peculiarities of human behavior on the subject matter. The wealth of information and trivia can sustain a long social conversation, or cut it short abruptly!

To 'Air' is Human Volume Two

AirVeda: Ancient & New Medical Wisdom, Digestion & Gas covers the remarkable advances in the understanding of digestive health and wellness. New information about the critical role of genomics, epigenetics, the gut microbiome, and the gut-brain-microbiome-diet axis are opening new avenues to optimal whole body health and wellness. An appreciation of the ancient wisdom of Ayurveda and other disciplines shows that they had advanced insights into the nature of the human body and the holistic approach. Although intestinal gas, basic bodily functions, and feces have been topics culturally suppressed, knowledge and understanding are needed to achieve and maintain optimal health. This volume, and others in the series, provide an informative and entertaining in depth look at the amazing world of human health and digestion.

"Ayurveda is a 5,000 year old system of natural healing that reminds us that health is the balanced and dynamic integration between our environment, body, mind and spirit. In Dr. Joseph Weiss' book, AirVeda, he provides an informative and entertaining approach to sharing insights about our digestive system and wellbeing by applying the ancient wisdom of Ayurveda to everyday life." **Deepak Chopra, MD**

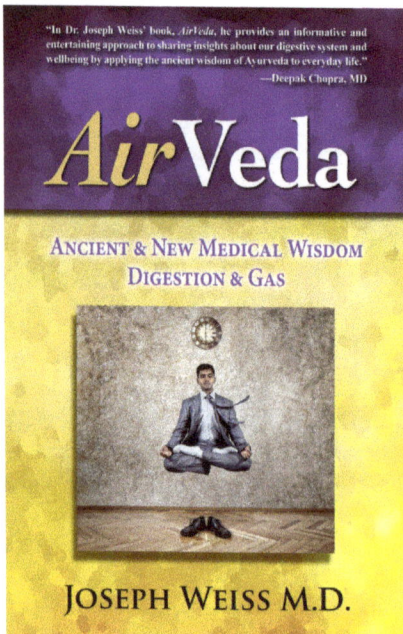

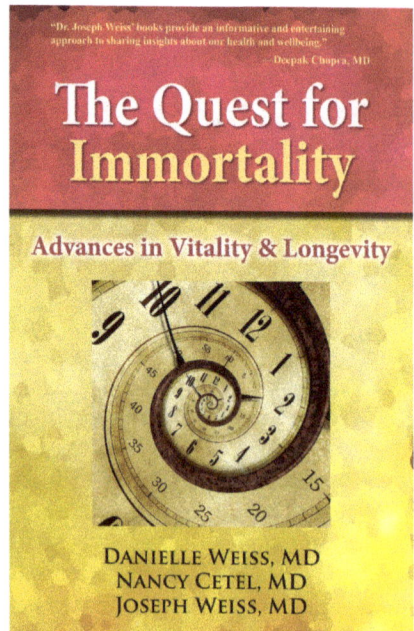

The Quest for Immortality, Advances in Vitality & Longevity provides an informative and enlightening overview of the remarkable advances in science and medicine that are dramatically enhancing human health and lifespan. The volume is written in clear, understandable, and engaging language with striking colorful illustrations. From groundbreaking nanotechnology to genomics and stem cells, the secrets of vitality and longevity are being uncovered along with more traditional advances and practical insights into disease prevention and health enhancement.

An even more comprehensive yet entertaining series are the extensive volumes of *Digestive Health & Disease, An Illustrated Encyclopedia of Everything You Ever Wanted To Know About Digestion & Nutrition*. These volumes are a uniquely informative, entertaining, and lavishly illustrated compendium of alimentary knowledge and eccentricities. It covers everything you ever wanted to know about digestion and nutrition in health and disease. Volumes One through Five are available on Amazon.com.

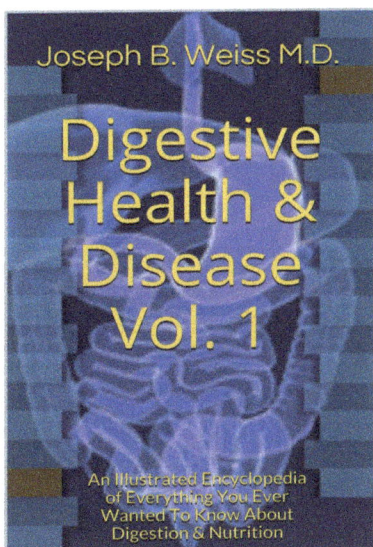

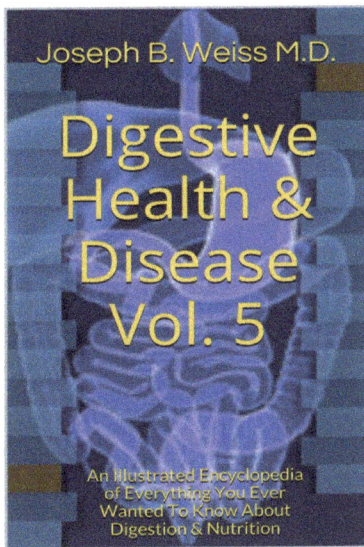

Organized as a reader friendly encyclopedia, the volumes cover over two thousand five hundred subject topics. Each volume may be utilized as an independent fully contained resource for the subjects it covers. The extensive size and scope of the series allows topics to be included that are rarely discussed in other books in the field and may be of great interest to the curious mind.

Written for the intelligent lay public, the medical and scientific terminology is translated into plain English. Practical and useful information and guidance are the primary goals, but entertaining and interesting information is included wherever possible. Designed for the visual learner as well, the clearly written text is supplemented by excellent photographs, illustrations, and charts. The reader will be informed, entertained, and the beneficiary of their newfound understanding of the universal process of digestion and metabolism that is the basis of all healthy living.

The website www.smartaskbooks.com has a complete list of books and programs by Joseph Weiss, MD, FACP, FACG, AGAF, Clinical Professor of Medicine (Gastroenterology), University of California, San Diego.

Appendix A: Colloquialism, Idiom, & Synonym of Fart

The word fart is one of the oldest words in the English language. One of the most important dictionaries in the long history of the language is Samuel Johnson's *A Dictionary of the English Language* published in 1755. An important innovation in his dictionary was the use of quotations from literature to illustrate the usage of the word defined.

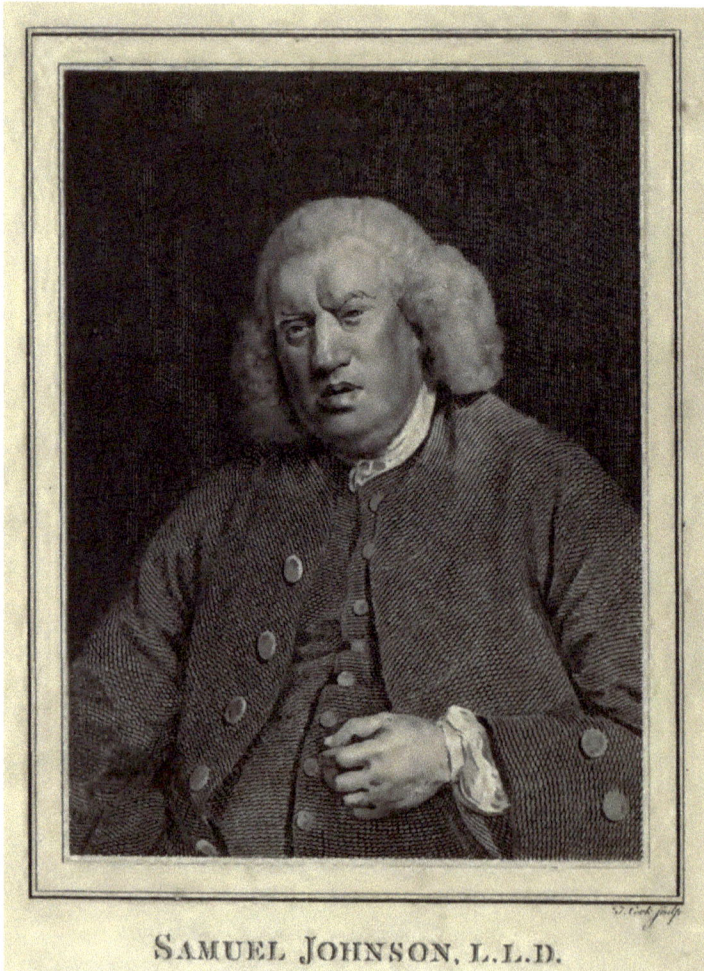

SAMUEL JOHNSON, L.L.D.

Public Domain

The word fart is proper English, and was in use for hundreds of years, before relatively recent polite and civil society considered it taboo. Without an alternative word, euphemisms were created and used. The number of terms that were synonymous with fart numbers in the many hundreds. The partial list that follows gives a good approximation of the wide variety of colorful alternatives.

FART. *n. f.* [ꝼeþꞇ, Saxon.] Wind from behind.

    Love is the *fart*
Of every heart;
It pains a man when 'tis kept clofe ;
And others doth offend, when 'tis let loofe. *Suckling.*
To FART. *v. a.* [from the noun.] To break wind behind.

    As when we a a gun difcharge,
Although the bore be ne'er fo large,
Before the flame from muzzle burft,
Juft at the breech it flafhes firft;
So from my lord his paffion broke,
He *farted* firft and then he fpoke.   *Swift.*

Public Domain

The origins of these phrases, and their acceptance into the cultural lexicon, are often obscured. Sometimes new words are added simply by an author creatively using a newly invented word in a literary work. I am fond of a new word coined by David Gilmour, an entrepreneur and philanthropist. He described a word that combines the sense of anticipation and subsequent disappointment, when the experience is not as satisfying as expected. The word he crated 'anticipointment' is a portmanteau that should stand the test of time.

I am tempted to add to new words to the lexicon as well. I am using the author's prerogative to place the words in print below, and although I have not heard them elsewhere before someone may well have created them before me. The first word is fartigenic, or its alternative, fartogenic. Fartigenic is a portmanteau combining the word fart with the Latin root suffix -genic of genesis and creation fame. The word describes a substance, which induces the creation of a fart. Refried beans and chili con carne would be good examples of fartigenic foods. My second word creation choice would be related to the common phrase stomach flu when used to describe a viral gastroenteritis with diarrhea and farting. We often use the term flu when describing a viral illness even though in is not a true influenza virus. I am taking poetic liberty to borrow the influenza root word to describe a stomach flu as 'inflatuenza'. My third and final word would be an alternative word for bloating or distention. As one could consider this condition to be caused by the retention and delay of the necessary intestinal gas passage, I suggest the word 'gastipated'. Okay, so maybe that word will not stand the test of time, and I should cease my word mining activities while I still have you as a reader.

What follows are the colloquialisms, idioms, and synonyms, that for better or for worse, are part of the lexicon.

A bit more choke and you would have started – an Australian phrase
    often addressed to the person responsible for an audible fart

Afflatus – Although it contains the word flatus this word has nothing
    to do with a fart. Flatus is Latin for a blowing, breathing, or a
    wind. Afflatus is a word first used by Cicero in his volume *De
    Natura Deorum* (*The Nature of the Gods*). In his book it is used as
    a phrase for a sudden rush of unexpected breath, a fresh
    inspiration. The word inspiration is derived from inspire, to
    breath as well as to have a creative thought or new idea. Afflatus
    thus can mean a divine inspiration. The only way to associate it
    with a fart is to consider it to be the exact opposite of a brain fart.

After thunder comes the rain – Phrase used when fart is passed just
    before urinating.

Air bagel – Fart

Air biscuit – Fart

Anal acoustics - Fart

Anal ahem - Fart

Anal audio - Fart

Anal salute - Fart

Anal volcano - Fart

Aqua fart - An underwater fart bubble, usually seen in the bathtub
    or swimming pool. The only way to clearly see an otherwise
    invisible fart.

Arse blast - Fart

Artsy Fartsy – Presented as art and culture but just as likely to be
    seen as pretentious, eccentric, eclectic, and unworthy of
    sophisticated cultural approval.

As much chance as a fart in a thunderstorm, windstorm, blizzard,
    hurricane, tornado, gale, etcetera - Means having no chance at all.

Ass blaster - Fart

Ass biscuit - Fart

Ass thunder - Fart

Ass whistle - Fart

Brain fart – Mental lapse, which usually results in an error while
    doing a repetitive activity.

Backdoor breeze - Fart

Backfire - Fart

Barking spiders - Fart

Bean blower - Fart

Blast off - Fart

Blowing a Raspberry (or Strawberry) – Imitating the sound of a fart

by exhaling through pursed lips, usually as a sign of derision. Also
known as a Bronx cheer.

Blowing the butt bugle - Fart

Blowing you a kiss - Fart

Bomber - Fart

Bottom blast - Fart

Bottom burp - Fart

Break wind - Fart

Breath of fresh air - Fart

Bronx cheer - Imitating the sound of a fart by exhaling through
pursed lips, usually as a sign of derision. Also known as a Blowing
a Raspberry or Strawberry.

Brown horn brass choir - Fart

Brown thunder - Fart

Bun shaker - Fart

Burnin' rubber - Fart

Buster - Fart

Busting ass - Fart

Butt bleat - Fart

Butt burp - Fart

Butt percussion - Fart

Butt trumpet - Fart

Butt tuba - Fart

Buttock bassoon - Fart

Cheek flapper - Fart

Cheesin' - Fart

Colonic calliope - Fart

Crack a rat - Fart

Crack one off - Fart

Crack splitters - Fart

Crop dusting - Farting while passing seated bystanders

Crowd splitter - Fart

Cut a stinker - Fart

Cut loose - Fart

Cut the cheese - Fart

Cut the wind - Fart

Death breath - Fart

Deflate - Fart

Drop a barking spider - Fart

Drop a bomb - Fart

Drop ass - Fart

Dutch oven – Farting under the blankets while in bed, then covering
up your bedmate to share the aroma.

Empty my tank - Fart

Eproctophilia – A fart fetish, the receiving of sexual pleasure and
arousal from the fart of another. The author James Joyce (see

separate entry) describes this fetish in letters published after his death.

Exploding bottom - Fart

Exterminate - Fart

Farst – Descriptive of a fast fart

Fart – (Foreign languages) – Unrelated to the English usage of the word, in the German and Scandinavian languages the word means speed, often used in speeding or speed control zones signs. in Danish a *fartcertifikate* means a trade certificate. In Norwegian a *fart plan* means a schedule. The Norwegian phrase *stå på fartin* pronounced as stop-a –fartin means ready to leave. Likewise, the phrase *farts måler* pronounced as fart smeller refers to a speedometer. In Swedish a speed bump is called a *farthinder*. *Fartlek* is speed training by running at alternate intervals of fast and slow paces. Likewise, if you travel on a Scandinavian marine vessel you may see the control of engine speed labeled as *half fart* and *full fart* for half speed and full speed respectively. Fart kontrol zones are speed zones. In Germany a similar word *fahrt* means a journey, trip, tour, or passage. It is often seen in signs that say *einfahrt* (sounds like in-fart) and *ausfahrt* (sounds like out-fart) denoting entrance and exit respectively. In Spanish and Portuguese *fart* means an excess of anything, especially a food. One of the richest deserts they offer is called a *farte*, which means a fruit tarte in Spain and usually a sugar almond or cream cake in Portugal. In Italy the word *farto* means mattress. In Hungarian *fartaj* means buttocks. In Poland if you want to buy a popular candy bar with a name that that means lucky you will be looking for a *Fart* bar.

Fartalito - Word for a small fart combining English and Spanish (Spanglish)

Fartable farter – An individual who can fart on command

Fart about – Waste time on silly or unnecessary activities

Fart absorption ratio – Humorous descriptive of the quantity of farts that a material can absorb and retain before the trapped gas escapes. Usually used to describe furniture such as a chair, sofa, ottoman, cushions, mattress, but can also be applied to rugs, carpets, clothing, etcetera.

Fart ache – Descriptive of a fart so potent that exposure to the fumes gives a headache. May also be used to describe pain after farting with anorectal disease such as fissures, abscess, fistula, hemorrhoids, and after delivery or surgery.

Fartachoo – A fart and sneeze occurring simultaneously

Fartacious – Ability to produce copious farts, either by volume or frequency.

Fartacrite – An individual who is hypocritical about farts, considering the farts of others as objectionable while their own farts are perfectly acceptable.

Fart addict – One who is obsessed with farting, usually used to describe an individual who produces farts in prodigious frequency and quantity.

Fartage - (French) Waxing of cross-country skis, unrelated to fart.

Fart against thunder – The fart equivalent of urinating (pissing) into the wind.

Fartagious – Contagious farting, often noted in preadolescent males.

Fartaholic – An individual who is described as being addicted to farting, often used to describe a husband.

Fart alarm – When the need to fart is misinterpreted as the need to defecate. Also when a baby's diaper is changed assuming a bowel movement occurred, only to find the diaper is empty as it was just a fart.

Fartalicious – A particularly attractive fart, either by acoustics, aroma, or quantity. Also may be used as a sarcastic compliment denoting that the taste of a food or drink was offensive.

Fart amnesty – A zone where unhindered farting is allowed without criticism or limitation. The zone is usually defined by the significant other, and may be in a remote location and different time zone.

Fart and dart – An individual who release a fart and quickly departs to let others experience their fart. Also known as fart and run.

Fart and flee – A practical joke, often executed spontaneously on releasing a fart in a crowded public place. The person immediately behind you is left standing in the aromatic wake of your fart, is assumed to be the culprit, and is the recipient of abhorrent glares from others.

Fart angels – Actively moving arms and legs in the same fashion as one makes snow angels by lying down in the snow. The activity is done in the standing mode to help circulate the air in the hope of dissipating the smell.

Fartanoid – A frantic sense of insecurity that an impending fart may allow the release of bowel contents.

Fartapalooza – A spasm of frequent, voluminous, and typically audacious farts over a short period of time. More often occurs following ingestion of a fart inducing meal, such as refried beans.

Fart app – An application for mobile phones and other electronic devices that reproduces sounds that imitate the various acoustic forms of the art of the fart.

Fart around – Waste time on silly or unnecessary activities

Fart arpeggio – A fart that changes tone at least twice so that three or more notes are produced during its course. A master of this technique was Joseph Pujol, known as Le Pétomane, during his performance career on the Moulin Rouge in Paris.

Fartarrhea – Similar to shart as a combination of shit and fart, but with diarrhea and fart. The fart often releases a mist of liquid feces, which soil the underwear or clothing if not released while on a toilet.

Fart arse – (British) To be stupid, farting or mucking around.

Fart art – Euphemism for abstract art appearance of soiling of underwear upon passing a particularly powerful fart that carried some organic fecal matter, mucus, or moisture. More common with a bout of dysentery or diarrhea.

Fart ass – Similar to smart-ass

Fart attack – Condition of pain related to intestinal gas, including intestinal gas in the pre-fart stage of bloating and distension. Play on words with similarity to heart attack, Unfortunately symptoms that suggest intestinal gas discomfort (fart attack) may actually be due to a heart condition (heart attack) and delay urgently needed medical care. In this situation a misdiagnosed fart/heart attack can be a true life threatening condition. A popular dark humor cartoon illustration shows a family member misinterpreting a cardiologist as saying that her spouse had a massive 'fart attack'

Fart baby – Descriptive term for abdominal bloating from intestinal gas, more noticeable in young thin women who develop visible distension that gives the impression of an early pregnancy.

Fart bag – A plastic or paper bag used to capture and seal in a fart, to be subsequently opened in the face of an unsuspecting victim.

Fart bellows – Farting under a blanket while in bed, and then trying to clear the fart by using the blanket as a bellow. The opposite of a Dutch oven, where the goal is to trap the fart under the blanket.

Fart blanche – To be given carte blanche to fart at will under the blanket or other locations.

Fart box – A euphemism for anus, rectum, and rectal cavity.

Fart brain – Used similarly to airhead, suggesting that farts rather than brains reside in the skull

Fart breath – Foul smelling breath

Fart bride – A woman who was very discrete about bodily functions, especially farts, before marriage, but loses all inhibitions after marriage.

Fart bubble – An underwater fart bubble, usually seen in the bathtub or swimming pool. The only way to clearly see an otherwise invisible fart.

Fart catcher – Nickname given to horsemen seated immediately behind the horses pulling a carriage. Also used to describe assistants and servants who walk a few paces behind them superior.

Fart buddy – A friend who is close enough that farting in their presence does not lead to any offense, and may contribute to an open farting atmosphere.

Fart burn – The burning rectal or anal sensation after extensive diarrhea and farting. Also may be experienced after eating hotly spiced foods.

Fart camouflage – Also known as fart camo. Making noise by an activity to hide the sound of a fart. The goal is to create a distraction to allow the noisy passage of a fart to go undetected. Using an air freshener, perfume, or other strong aroma may be used in an attempt to mask the smell. Opening windows and doors with the excuse that it is too warm is often used as a fart camouflage maneuver.

Fart candy – Candy that induces farting by having a high content of non-absorbable sugars. Dietetic candies often have this property.

Fart door - Colloquial term for anus.

Farter – A person who procrastinates by farting around. (British) Slang term for anus, also a sleeping bag which is warmed by farts.

Farterbox – (Irish) Slang for anus

Fartface – Facial expression that gives the impression that the wearer is smelling a noxious fart. Also slang for an idiot or stupid person.

Fart factory – Slang for anus, also to describe a frequent or voluminous farter.

Fart fetish – Formally known as eproctophilia, the receiving of sexual pleasure and arousal from the fart of another. The author James Joyce (see separate entry) describes this fetish in letters published after his death.

Farther, Farthest, Farthermost – These words denote greater distance from an object, an are unrelated to the word fart that is contained within their spelling. The only way they may be tied to the word fart is in vocabulary games like Scrabble, Boggle, and others where additional points may be gained by adding letters to a core word.

Fart higher than your ass – Arrogant and pretentious, translation of original phrase from the French *péter plus haut que son cul.*

Farthing – British coin currency with a nominal value. Benjamin Franklin uses the nominal currency as a double entendre at the end of his proposal to the Royal Academy of Brussels to create an award for an additive that word give farts a pleasant smell (see entry on Benjamin Franklin)

Farthingale – A hoop like structure worn under the skirt by women in the late 16th and early 17th centuries to give it the shape of a bell or cone. Originally introduced at the Spanish court it subsequently became popular fashion in Tudor England. Although the shape and structure may have been helpful to muffle the sound and contain the aroma of a fart, there is no evidence that the name was related to the word fart. One theory behind the development of the farthingale was to hide a pregnancy that may have resulted from illicit relationships.

Fart in a bottle – Description of restless movement suggestive of agitation or being flustered.

Fart in a thunderstorm or windstorm –Figure of speech suggesting the event is unnoticed or unidentifiable because of background activity. When in the phrase as much chance as a fart in a thunderstorm, windstorm, blizzard, hurricane, tornado, gale, etc. it means having no chance at all.

Farting clapper - Anus, or more pejorative asshole.

Farting fanny – Nickname given to heavy German artillery guns used during World War I

Farting shot – An action designed to show contempt.

Farting through silk –financially affluent, able to afford luxuries

Fart lighting – Ignition of flammable gas (methane and/or hydrogen) released in some farts. Serious injury and burns have resulted from this activity, most often seen in adolescent males.

Fartman – A fictional superhero popularized by television and radio personality Howard Stern (see separate entry).

Fart monkey – Term of endearment, usually for a pet such as a dog or cat that farts whenever it needs to. The fart monkey can also serve as fart camouflage and be designated as the source of an errant fart.

Fart sucker – A parasite or toady willing to do whatever it takes to curry favor. Analogous to ass kisser, brown-nose equivalent. Interesting tie in to French slang for criminal suspect. The French pronounce suspect as soos-pay, the same way they would pronounce the words *sucé pet*, which translates literally as fart sucker. The French authorities can use the double entendre to express their dislike of a suspect without being chastised.

Fart time – Describes employed hours per week that fall between full-time and part-time employment. Usually defined as between twenty-one and thirty-five hours of work time per week.

Fire a stink torpedo - Fart

Fire the retro-rocket - Fart

Firing scud missiles - Fart

Fizzler - Fart

Flamethrower - Fart

Flamer - Fart

Flapper - Fart

Flatulate - Fart

Flatulence - Fart

Flatus - Fart

Flipper - Fart

Float an air biscuit - Fart

Floof - Fart

Fluffy - Fart

Fog slicer - Fart
Fowl howl - Fart
Fragrant fuzzy - Fart
Free-floating anal vapors - Fart
Free Jacuzzi - Fart
Freep - Fart
Frequency Actuated Rectal Tremor - Fart
Fumigate - Fart
Funky rollers - Fart
Gas attack - Fart
Gas blaster - Fart
Gas from the ass - Fart
Gas master - Fart
Gaseous intestinal by-products – Fart
Ghost turd - Fart
Grandpa - Fart
Gravy pants - Fart
Great brown cloud - Fart
Heinus anus - Fart
Hole flappage - Fart
Hole flapper - Fart
Honk - Fart
HUMrrhoids - Fart
Hydrogen bomb - Fart
Ignition - Fart
Insane in the methane - Fart
Invert a burp - Fart
Jet propulsion - Fart
Joan of Fart – Artful nickname for a female who has farted audibly
    or aromatically.
Jockey burner - Fart
Jumping guts - Fart
Just calling your name - Fart
Just keeping warm - Fart
Just the noise - Fart
Kaboom - Fart
K-Fart - Fart
Kill the canary - Fart
Lay a wind loaf - Fart
Lay an air biscuit - Fart
Leave a gas trap - Fart
Let a beefer - Fart
Let a brewer's fart – To have diarrhea.
Let each little bean be heard - Fart
Let one fly - Fart
Let one go - Fart

Let the beans out - Fart
Lethal cloud - Fart
Letting one rip - Fart
Lingerer - Fart
Made a gas blast – Fart
Make a stink - Fart
Make a trumpet of one's ass – Fart
Mating call of the barking spider - Fart
Meteor – Fart
Methane bomb - Fart
Methane production experiment - Fart
Moon gas - Fart
Mud duck - Fart
Must be a sewer around - Fart
Nose death - Fart
Odor bubble - Fart
Odorama - Fart
Old fart – An old man, a person in authority very set in their ways, inflexible.
One-man jazz band - Fart
One-gun salute - Fart
Painting the elevator - Fart
Pant stainer - Fart
Panty burp - Fart
Parp - Fart
Party in your pants - Fart
Pass gas - Fart
Pass wind - Fart
Pet – Fart (French) The diminutive for fart in the French language. It makes the written English use of pet shop, pet food, love of pets, etc. an interesting translation. The pronunciation is different however, as pet is pronounced as pay in French
Pissed as a fart – Very drunk (British & Australian)
Play the tuba - Fart
Playing the trouser tuba - Fart
Plotcher (aka a wet one) – Fart
Poof - Fart
Poop gas - Fart
Poot - Fart
Pootie – Fart
Pop - Fart
Pop a fluffy - Fart
Preventing spontaneous human combustion – Fart
Puff, the magic dragon - Fart
Quack - Fart
Raspberry (Razz) - Slang for *'blowing a raspberry or strawberry'*,

imitating the sound of a fart by exhaling through pursed lips, usually as a sign of derision. Also known as a Bronx cheer.

Rebuild the ozone layer one poof at a time - Fart

Rectal honk - Fart

Rectal shout - Fart

Rectal tremor - Fart

Release a squeaker - Fart

Release an ass biscuit - Fart

Release gas - Fart

Rep - Fart

Rimshot - Fart

Rip ass - Fart

Rip one - Fart

Ripple fart - Fart

Roast the Jockeys - Fart

Rotting vegetation - Fart

Royal fart – A fart of unusual distinction.

Safety - Fart

Salute your shorts - Fart

SAS (silent and scentless) – Fart

SBD (silent but deadly) – Fart

Set off an SBD - Fart

Shart – Fart passage that allows the escape of fecal material. The word shart is a portmanteau of shit and fart.

Shit fumes - Fart

Shit honker - Fart

Shit vapor - Fart

Shoot the cannon - Fart

Shoppin' at Wal-Fart - Fart

Silent and scentless (SAS) – Fart

Silent but deadly (SBD) – Fart

Singe the carpet - Fart

Singing the anal anthem - Fart

Sounding the sphincter scale - Fart

Sound of a barking spider - Fart

Sound of a wompus cat - Fart

Sparrow-fart - Denotes the earliest of daylight, early dawn, sunrise, sunup, first light of day. Although it uses the same word 'fart' it is not a reference to the passage of intestinal gas

Sphincter song - Fart

Spit a brick - Fart

Squeak one out - Fart

Squeaker - Fart

Steamer - Fart

Step on a duck - Fart

Step on a frog - Fart

To 'Air' is Human Volume Two

Stink bomb - Fart
Stink burger - Fart
Strangling the stank monkey - Fart
Strawberry - Slang for imitating the sound of a fart by exhaling
    through pursed lips, usually as a sign of derision. Also known as a
    Bronx cheer or a raspberry
Stress release - Fart
Tail wind - Fart
The colonic calliope - Fart
The dog did it - Fart
The F bomb - Fart
The gluteal tuba - Fart
The Sound and the Fury - Fart
The stink's gone into the fabric - Fart
The third state of matter - Fart
The toothless one speaks - Fart
Thunder pants - Fart
Thunderspray - Fart
Toilet tune - Fart
Toot - Fart
Toot your own horn - Fart
Trelblow - Fart
Triple flutter blast - Fart
Trouser cough - Fart
Trouser trumpet - Fart
Turd honking - Fart
Turd hooties - Fart
Turn on the air conditioning in the colon - Fart
Uncorked symphony - Fart
Under burp - Fart
Venting one - Fart
Wet one - Fart
What the dog did - Fart
Who Cut the Cheese - Fart
Wrong way burping - Fart
Zinger – Fart

Appendix B: Fart in Foreign Languages

American Sign Language:

The non-dominant hand is an "A" or an "S" handshape. The dominant hand is a bent hand and is held so that the fingers are underneath the pinkie side of the non-dominant "fist." The dominant hand "unbends" and bends one time as if showing gas escaping. Here is a "one handed" version of fart, both versions are widely used. You start by opening up the pinkie, and then the ring and middle finger. The index finger stays curled up. Then you reverse and close the middle, then ring, then pinkie fingers. For comic effect or emphasis you can puff one cheek and force a bit of air through your lips at the corner of your mouth.

Afrikaans: fart
Albanian: pordhÃ«, pjerdh; pordhë, hajvan, pjerdh
Arabic: ضرطة, نفخة ضرط, ضرطة , ha ridge
Armenian: fart, basz toe
Avestan: pərəδaiti
Azerbaijani: osurmaq
Basque: fart
Belarusian: Ð¿ÐµÑ€Ð´ÐµÑ‚ÑŒ
Bulgaria: fart Флатуленция, пръдня
Catalan: pet, *colloq* pet, *colloq* torracollons, *colloq* tirar-se un pet,
    fer-se un pet
Chinese (Simplified): 屁, 放屁 屁 fom pee/ pie Chee
Chinese (Traditional): 屁, 放屁 屁 fom pee/ pie Chee
Croatian: prdnuti, vjetar, prdac, ispuštati vjetrove, prditi
Czech: prd
Danish: prut
Dutch: wind laten, winderigheid, een wind laten, een scheet laten,
    (slang) scheet (slang)
Esperanto: furzi, furzo
Estonian: pieru
Farsi: gooz bede, گوز، گوزیدن
Filipino: umut-ot, kabag-gas oh mo toot ka
Finnish: pieru
French: péter, pet, dis gas, péter (argot); lâcher une vesse; vesser pet
    (argot), vesse, merdeux
Galician: peidar
Georgian: fart
German: furz, flatulenz, fuhren sie gas, furzen, sich mit jedem dreck
    abgeben (Umgangsprache), scheißer (slang)
Greek: πέρδομαι (perdomai), ÎºÎ»Î½Î¿, κλάνω, πέρδομαι κλανιά,
    πορδή
Haitian Creole: fart
Hebrew: "סלנג) "נאד, נפיחה (סלנג) "נאד לתקוע", "להפליץ)

311

Hindi: पादना

Hmong: tso paus, tawb paus

Hungarian: fing, fingik, szellentés

Icelandic: rÃ¦fill

Ilokano: uttot

Indonesian: kentut

Irish: fart

Italian: fart, flatulenza, pass il gas, scoreggiare scoreggio, peto

Japanese: おなら, 屁, おならをする, 屁をこく（俗語）おなら, 屁（俗語）

Korean: 방귀 뀌다, bung koo

Latin: pēdĕre

Latvian: fart

Lithuanian: bezdalius

Macedonia: Ð¿Ñ€Ð´ÐµÐ¶

Malay: kentut

Maltese: fart

Norwegian: fart

Persian: گوز, گُز، گوزیدن گوز gooz bede

Philippine: kabag-gas, oh mo toot ka, umut-ot,

Polish: bpierd, pierdzieÄ‡, gazy jelitowe, parvee etra, vi pierdzieć, pierdnięcie, pierdnąć

Portuguese: peidar, pedo, flatulência, soltar um pum (gíria) peido,

Romanian: bÃ¢Å¾i, flatulenţă, gaze (vulgar), vint, a da vinturi,

Russian: пердеть (perdet'), издавать громкий треск, пукнуть громкий треск при выходе газов из организма, непристойный звук; пукание; старик зря терять время Ð¿ÐµÑ€Ð´ÐµÑ‚ÑŒ, метеоризм, puk nee
The Russian words for fart include *perdyozh* (first act of breaking wind), *perdun* (perpetrator and outcome), *perdil'nik* (place from where it comes), *Perun* (ancient God of wind), *bzdun* (silent fart), *bzdyukha* (silent fart as well as a stupid jerk). Some of the Russian verbs for the action of farting are particularly colorful. *Perdet'* (to fart with or without sound), *bzdet'* (to fart silently), *pereperdet* (to fart repeatedly), and my favorite word *nabzdet'sya* (ton fart silently to one's complete and utter satisfaction!).

Sanskrit: pardate

Serbian: Ð¿Ñ€Ð½ÑƒÑ‚Ð¸

Slovak: prd

Slovenian: prdec

Somali: doughso

Spanish: pedo, tirarse un pedo (familismo), peo, pasar gasses, peer, ventosear, ventoseo, cuesco

Swahili: fart, kyfoosi

Swedish: fart, fjärt , flatulens, prutta, fjärta (slang) prutt, fjärt (slang)

Tagalog (Philippine): kabag-gas, oh mo toot ka, umut-ot,
Taiwanese: 放屁 屁 funkee-pass gas
Thai: ตด, ฟาท, ลมตด (ผายลม),ตด,การผายลม,บตก,ผายลม
Turkish: osuruk, ul cer, osurmak, gaz yapmak osuruk, yellenme
Urdu: سڑنا باؤ -مارنا پهسـكـي يا پاد -پادنا ,گوز -باؤ -پهسـكـي -پاد ,گوز
Vietnamese: đánh rắm, trung tiện, dit, danh từ, đùi 0 rắm,
    nội động từ, chùi gháu
Visayan: otot
Welsh: basio gwynt
Yiddish: פֿאָרצן

Index (including Volume One)

To 'Air' is Human Volume Two

www.ingramcontent.com/pod-product-compliance
Lightning Source LLC
Chambersburg PA
CBHW051245020426
42333CB00025B/3066